7-INGREDIENT
HEALTHY PREGNANCY
COOKBOOK

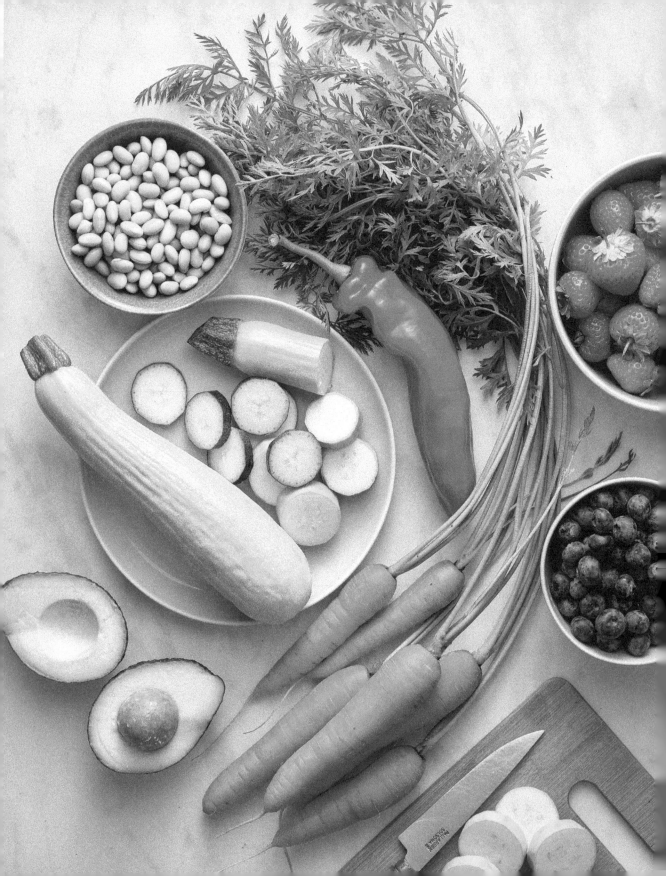

7-INGREDIENT
HEALTHY
PREGNANCY
COOKBOOK

75 EASY RECIPES FOR EVERY STAGE OF PREGNANCY

LAUREN MANAKER, MS, RDN, LDN, CLEC

PHOTOGRAPHY BY DARREN MUIR

ROCKRIDGE PRESS

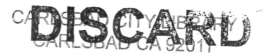

Cover Designer: Amanda Kirk; Interior Designer: Irene Vandervoort
Art Producer: Janice Ackerman
Editor: Annie Choi
Production Editor: Jenna Dutton
Production Manager: Sandy Noman
Cover: Grilled Chicken, Avocado, and Mango Salad, page 54

Photography ©2021 Darren Muir. Food styling by Yolanda Muir.

Paperback ISBN: 978-1-64876-344-1 | eBook ISBN: 978-1-63807-282-9
R0

JUL 2 0 2022

This book is dedicated to all of the tired parents-to-be who are trying their very best.

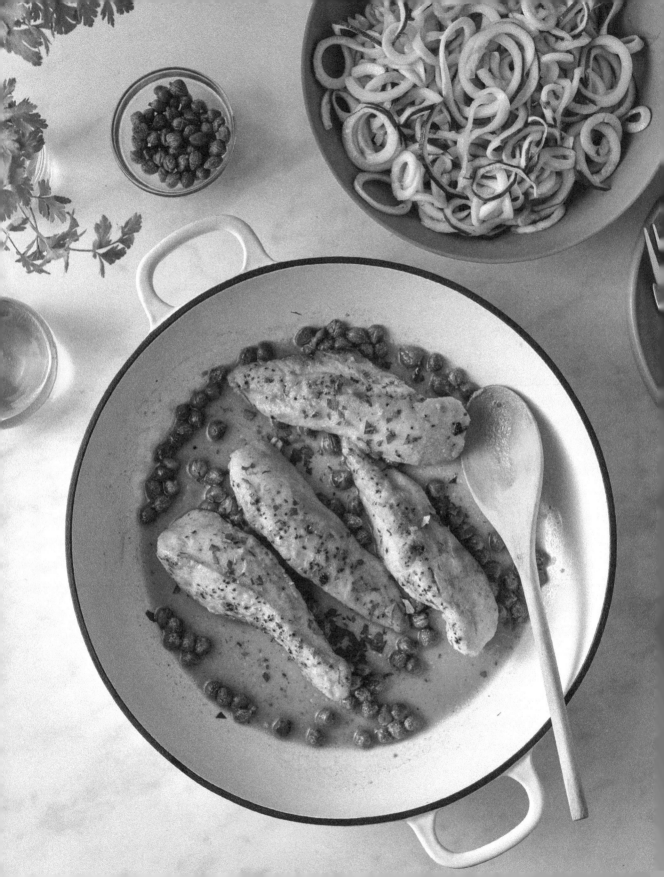

CONTENTS

CHICKEN PICCATA
WITH ZOODLES (PAGE 94)

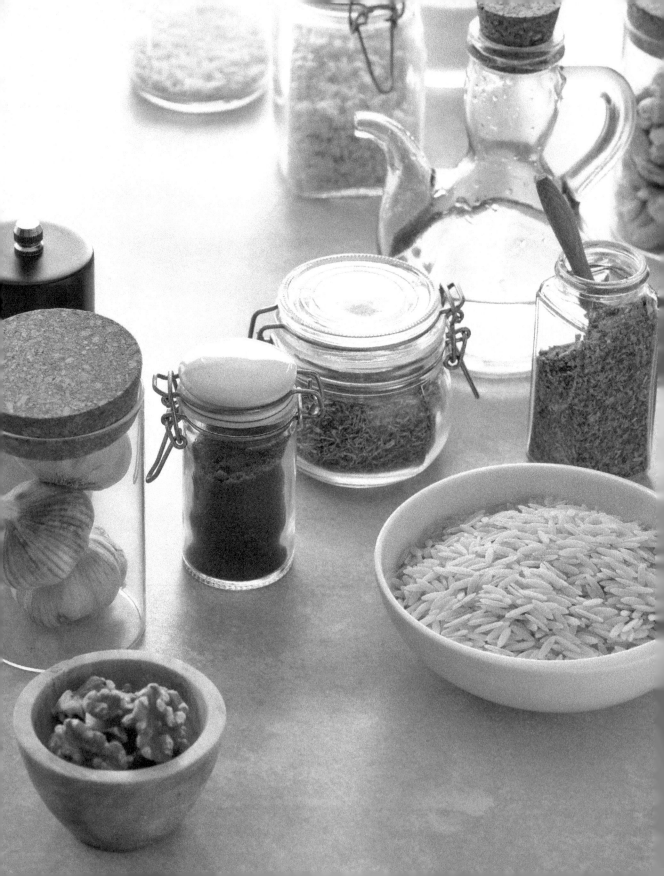

INTRODUCTION

Congratulations on your pregnancy! Expecting a child, whether it's your first or your third, is a joyful and exciting experience, but it can also be nerve-wracking and exhausting. With so many things running through your mind during these next nine months (ahem, next 18 years), the last thing you have time for is thinking about what the heck you're going to eat! That's where I come in.

I am a registered dietitian and mother to a fantastic little girl. When I was pregnant, I found a slew of "pregnancy-friendly" recipes online that required a laundry list of ingredients, had complicated instructions, and took way too long to cook. I would occasionally buy the ingredients for certain recipes with the best of intentions, but more often than not, I would resort to a sandwich and a bowl of soup because I was too tired and busy to whip up a complicated meal.

I understand that knowing what to eat while pregnant can be a lot to think about, and that's why I believe in this simple, ingredients-focused approach. As a prenatal registered dietitian-nutritionist, I have created these recipes to take the guesswork out of eating for two. Best of all, the recipes have seven main ingredients or fewer, which means cooking healthy meals can be easier than getting in your car and snagging some take-out—and you'll be getting all the nutrients you need for a healthy, happy pregnancy.

This book puts 75 simple and nourishing recipes at your fingertips. But you will also get a pregnancy superfoods chart; meal plans to address nausea, low energy, and swelling; and substitution tips for swapping out ingredients that don't agree with you. As a bonus, I've even included instructions on how to make your own homemade belly butter!

With these recipes and helpful tips, eating well while pregnant is not only possible but easy. Thank you for allowing me to be a part of your journey.

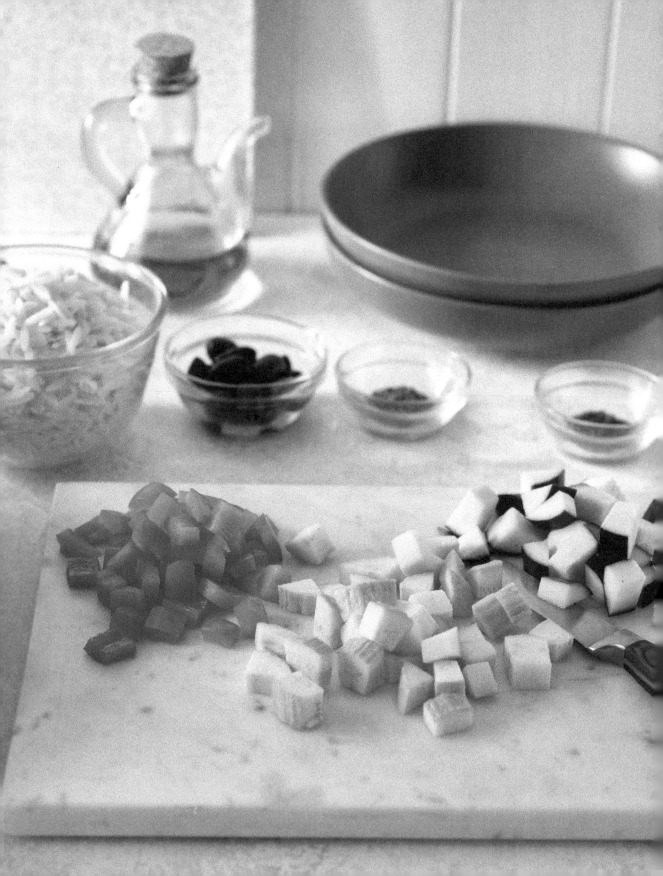

ONE

A HEALTHY, HAPPY PREGNANCY

The recipes and advice in this cookbook make it easy for you to nourish yourself and your baby with key nutrients that support a healthy pregnancy.

In this chapter, you will get an overview of eating well when you are eating for two. While this is a cookbook first and foremost, I suggest you familiarize yourself with this nutrition information so you can make the best decisions for your growing baby.

What Does Nutritious Eating Look Like During Pregnancy?

When a person becomes pregnant, they often instinctually understand that they should be eating a healthy and balanced diet. After all, everything the pregnant person eats is essentially what the baby eats, too.

But knowing that you *should* eat well and knowing *how* to eat well are two different things, and they don't always go hand in hand. That's where this guide comes in, helping you navigate how to eat well so you are providing yourself and your baby with the best forms of nourishment and helping you feel as comfortable and energized as possible in the process.

There is no one way to eat healthily while pregnant—yes, there are some more or less hard-and-fast rules (for example, limiting alcohol and caffeine, fast food, and heavily processed foods), but there are many different paths to getting the nutrition you and your baby need.

A great rule of thumb is to listen to your body. If a certain food doesn't sound or feel good to eat, don't force yourself to eat it! And if all your body wants is a smoothie, that's fine, too. Every pregnancy journey is different, and every pregnancy diet is different. As long as you are including nutrient-dense foods and high-quality prenatal supplements in your plan, you will be nourishing your baby during pregnancy.

If all you can handle is grab-and-go (for instance, if you're too nauseated to eat a traditional meal or you're juggling a job and older kids), there are some ways to make smaller meals, smoothies, and even snacks into nutritious powerhouses.

There is a lot of information floating around the internet that is focused on prenatal nutrition, and unfortunately, most of it can sound overwhelming. Rest assured that, by reading this book, you can stop frantically scrolling for information. Take solace knowing that you have a dietitian-approved cookbook in your hands that will help you get what you need without the fuss.

What to Expect . . .

In this section, you will learn all about general nutritional recommendations for supporting a healthy pregnancy (and your growing baby) and what pregnancy symptoms you can expect, especially as they relate to food. While I will give you some specific guidelines in this section and chapter, it is imperative to be mindful of a few guidelines that should be followed throughout your pregnancy, like staying hydrated, taking prenatal vitamin supplements, getting adequate calories, and eating nutrient-dense foods.

Each trimester comes with its own unique nutrition needs due to the baby's stage of development. Here is a brief guide of what you can expect in each of the three trimesters.

IN YOUR FIRST TRIMESTER

During the first few months of your pregnancy, your baby is already starting to grow and develop. Since the neural tube is beginning to form, it's crucial that you take in adequate amounts of folic acid or folate, vitamin B_{12}, and choline to support healthy formation during the first stage of your journey. Eating foods like leafy green veggies, oranges, egg yolks, and chicken can be great sources of these key nutrients.

The brain and eyes are in the beginning stages of development, too. DHA, a nutrient primarily found in oily fish, plays a pivotal role in brain and eye development during pregnancy, and should be a focus during this trimester. If you can't stomach a piece of fish, a DHA supplement should be in your arsenal (algae-based options are available for those following a vegan diet).

You may start to feel a bit queasy and totally exhausted during this stage. That is totally normal; in many cases, these symptoms go away once you reach your second trimester.

IN YOUR SECOND TRIMESTER

During your second trimester, your baby is continuing to develop, and your belly will likely grow as a result. Many of the pesky symptoms of early pregnancy should subside, but unfortunately, that is not the case for everybody.

Starting in your second trimester, it's important to pay attention to your iron and calcium intake. Your iron needs increase to 27 mg/day during this stage. If your prenatal vitamin does not contain iron, you want to make sure you are eating iron-rich foods like lean red meat, certain shellfish, and dark leafy greens. You'll also need adequate calcium to support your little one's growing bones. Dairy foods, almonds, and tofu are natural sources of calcium.

As your belly and your baby both grow, you want to make sure that you are not only eating the right foods but also that you are also eating enough. Your calorie and protein needs also typically increase by the second trimester; however, your specific requirements will vary based on factors like your pre-pregnancy weight and how many babies you are carrying.

Finally, don't forget about hydration. Drinking enough fluid is critical to help support your growing belly. Free of sugar, calories, and caffeine, water is always your best bet.

IN YOUR THIRD TRIMESTER

During the home stretch of your pregnancy, your baby is growing and growing (and growing!). Organs continue to develop, and your baby looks more like a little human instead of a little tadpole.

Even though your belly is getting larger, and you may not feel hungry, it is important to continue to eat nutrient-dense foods. Fiber will be your best friend if you are feeling constipated—a condition that is very common at this stage as your hormones can do a number on your digestive system.

Key nutrients continue to be important during this final stage of your pregnancy, including DHA omega-3 fatty acids, iron, calcium, and iodine (a nutrient that supports a baby's brain development). Although many organs will have developed by the end of your pregnancy, it is still important to support your body and your baby by taking in nutrient-dense foods, especially if you are planning on breastfeeding.

IN YOUR FOURTH TRIMESTER

Your fourth trimester is the first three months postpartum—a time when the baby is adjusting to its new world and your body is managing hormonal and physical changes.

Regardless of how you delivered your baby, your body went through something major to bring a tiny human into the world. Thus, supporting your body for a successful recovery is of the utmost importance. And while eating your favorite snacks like cookies and ice cream is fine on occasion, fitting in foods that help your body recover should be the priority.

Foods that contain high-quality protein (like meats, dairy, beans, and nuts), vitamin C (like citrus foods and strawberries), and choline (like egg yolks, chicken, and peanuts) are all excellent additions to your postpartum diet plan.

If you are breastfeeding, your calorie needs are even higher now than when you were pregnant. Having nutrient-dense snacks and the ingredients for easy meals ready to go will be your lifeline. Foods like hard-boiled eggs, oatmeal, and peanut butter on whole-grain crackers are great choices to keep on hand.

WHAT TO DO WHEN
YOU JUST DON'T FEEL LIKE EATING

Whether it is due to nausea, exhaustion, or the baby pressing up against your stomach, lack of appetite can happen during pregnancy.

If you simply don't feel like eating, know that full-blown meals are not necessary 100 percent of the time. Here are some simple ways to ensure you're getting the nutrition you need without causing yourself added discomfort.

EAT SMALL MEALS THROUGHOUT THE DAY: Once you've found a few nutritious snacks that you can tolerate even when feeling nauseated, schedule snack breaks throughout the day with these foods. Eating a little something every two hours is good practice.

SIP ON SMOOTHIES: Blending foods like greens, cauliflower, and even sweet potatoes can help you meet your nutrition needs in a few simple sips.

KEEP GINGER HANDY: Ginger can ease an upset stomach and keep nausea at bay. Add fresh ginger to smoothies or meals or suck on a ginger candy to help settle your stomach.

TAKE PRENATAL VITAMINS WITH FOOD: While prenatal vitamins continue to be an important part of your pregnancy diet, some can be tough on your stomach. Taking your vitamin with food or before bed helps ease stomach upset. In some cases, you may need to change vitamin brands. Gummy vitamins can be a temporary fix until you start feeling better. Prenatal vitamin changes should always be discussed with your health-care provider.

GO FOR A WALK: Movement can help stimulate your appetite. If you are feeling like nothing belongs in your stomach, a quick stroll around the block may help kick-start your appetite.

TALK TO YOUR HEALTH-CARE PROVIDER: If you are having a hard time keeping food down or are truly not able to eat, consult your health-care provider to make sure you don't have major nutritional gaps. Be open with your provider and listen to their suggestions. It is important to take a proactive approach to your nutrition.

Optimal Nutrition with 7 Main Ingredients

Proper nutrition is the cornerstone of a healthy pregnancy, but some people may lead you to believe that cooking everything from scratch in complicated and time-consuming ways is necessary. That's simply not true. Whether you are juggling a demanding job, managing other kids, or simply don't want to spend your days toiling in the kitchen, you can absolutely meet your nutrition needs with easy dishes that focus on key ingredients.

Eating healthy during pregnancy is not about packing in all the nutrients all at once, but rather focusing on the most impactful, nutrient-dense ingredients for pregnancy support. **Toward that end, every recipe in this book contains no more than seven main ingredients, excluding a handful of staples you're likely to always have on hand: water or ice, salt, pepper, cooking spray, and oil (extra-virgin olive oil and coconut oil).**

In a nutshell, seven-ingredient recipes are a dream come true because:

- They are easier (and more cost-effective) to prepare, so they are doable even when you're low on energy.

- The focus is on getting the best quality of ingredients, not quantity—it's just the good stuff and nothing more.

- This way of cooking makes for a direct route to optimal prenatal nutrition.

Foods to Love during Pregnancy and Postpartum

When you are eating for a healthy pregnancy, it is refreshing to know that there aren't many foods that are totally restricted. Besides abiding by food safety precautions like avoiding undercooked foods, unpasteurized cheese, and alcoholic drinks, there aren't any foods that you have to completely forego during your next nine months. However, there are some dietitian-approved "superfoods" that pack a huge nutrition punch for pregnancy. Note that this list is not exhaustive and eating these foods won't guarantee a perfect pregnancy, but ideally these foods will show up on your plate more often than not. (See the Find Your

Pregnancy Superfood chart on page 9 for specific nutrients that can help relieve specific symptoms.)

DAIRY: Dairy, such as yogurt and pasteurized cheeses, provides a protein boost to your meals, but there aren't many foods that are packed with as many nutrients as good old-fashioned milk. In addition to calcium, milk contains vitamin D, magnesium, iodine, and many other nutrients. Sipping on a cold glass of milk is a simple way to get in some high-quality protein and key nutrients when you don't have an appetite.

DARK LEAFY GREENS: In general, dark leafy greens, like kale, spinach, and chard, are important to include in your prenatal diet because of their folate content. Adequate folate is needed to develop your baby's brain and spinal cord. Leafy greens also contain vitamin K, B vitamins, antioxidants, vitamin C, magnesium, and potassium. Many people find that the easiest way to get their greens is in a smoothie, which may help during times of severe nausea.

DRIED FRUIT: When you're craving a taste of something sweet, just a little dried fruit, like raisins, prunes, and dates, can go a long way. Not only will these little gems help satisfy your sweet tooth, but they are also packed with dietary fiber that will help combat constipation. They also contain iron that may help fight fatigue. Just make sure to choose options that aren't made with added sugars, and if you're sensitive to it, avoid dried fruits that contain sulfur dioxide.

EGGS: Choline is a key nutrient that pregnant people need in large quantities to help support baby's brain and spinal cord development. Unfortunately, there aren't too many foods that contain this nutrient in large amounts. Eggs, and specifically egg yolks, are unique because they not only contain around 150 mg of this brain-boosting nutrient, but they also contain other pregnancy-boosting vitamins and minerals, like iodine, vitamin B_{12}, and lutein.

EXTRA-VIRGIN OLIVE OIL: Loaded with healthy fats, antioxidants, and compounds that help combat inflammation, extra-virgin olive oil is a natural fat source that goes well with a slew of ingredients.

FRESH FRUITS AND VEGETABLES: Eating a variety of vegetables daily is crucial to a healthy pregnancy. They provide fiber and a veritable treasure trove of vitamins, minerals, and antioxidants. Avocados are a pregnancy favorite, and for good reason. They're low in sugar and naturally contain fiber, folate, and magnesium. Avocados can also help with morning sickness, fatigue, muscle cramps, and constipation. A few other superstars include berries, broccoli, citrus, and tomatoes.

GINGER: Known for its ability to offer nausea relief, including this natural root in your pregnancy diet may be the ticket to morning sickness relief.

LEAN MEAT: Mild-flavored cuts of chicken are a great source of lean protein, B vitamins, choline, and zinc, especially on days when it's hard to get other protein sources down. Lean beef, like flank steak, is a source of two extremely important pregnancy nutrients—iron and zinc. The high-quality protein that lean beef provides will serve any pregnant belly well, especially as your baby starts growing.

LEGUMES: Legumes, like black beans, chickpeas, and lentils, are wonderful sources of plant-based protein, fiber, iron, and antioxidants. They are also rich in folate, which is essential for a baby's neural tube development.

OILY FISH: Many experts recommend eating a low-mercury oily fish like salmon two times a week during pregnancy. Salmon is also a favorite because it is a high-quality source of protein and provides a slew of other key nutrients that both you and your baby need. Salmon is another great food to enjoy if you are managing gestational diabetes, as the healthy fats may help manage inflammation and blood sugar stabilization.

NUTS AND SEEDS: Nuts (especially walnuts) provide fiber and plant-based proteins. Seeds are also a great addition to your diet; chia seeds in particular are a standout. A natural source of healthy fats, calcium, and iron, they have many benefits, including constipation relief, and are also a fantastic addition to a gestational diabetes diet.

WHOLE GRAINS: Whole grains will give you energy while also providing essential nutrients like fiber, iron, and B vitamins. Good choices include oats and the superstar of superstars: quinoa. Quinoa is a complete source of protein and also contains notable amounts of fiber and iron, as well as potassium, magnesium, and even zinc.

FIND YOUR PREGNANCY SUPERFOOD

KEY NUTRIENT	BENEFITS	SUPERFOODS TO EAT	RECIPES
Calcium	Supports healthy bones and teeth	Chia seeds, cheese, figs, kefir, milk, tofu, yogurt	Chia Zinger (page 118), Papaya Chia Pudding (page 31), Ginger Tofu Citrus Bowl (page 80), Breakfast Parfait with Tahini, Maple Syrup, and Figs (page 26), Banana Kefir Shake (page 41)
Choline	Supports a baby's brain and spinal cord development	Cauliflower, chicken, egg yolks, peanuts, quinoa	Egg Drop Soup (page 73), Cauliflower and Potato Mash (page 60), Chicken and Quinoa Casserole with Broccoli (page 86)
DHA Omega-3 Fatty acids	Crucial to a baby's brain development	Salmon, shrimp	Salmon Salad with Dates (page 55), Walnut-Crusted Salmon (page 92)
Folic Acid/ Folate	Supports a baby's neural tube development	Avocado, leafy green veggies, legumes, nuts and seeds, oranges	Fizzy Citrus Cooler (page 101), Sweet Greens Smoothie (page 36), Chocolate Cranberry Bark (page 106)
Iodine	Supports a baby's brain development	Cheese, eggs, milk, nori (seaweed), shrimp	Miso and Veggie Soup (page 75), PB&J French Toast (page 27)
Iron	May help combat pregnancy fatigue and help reduce the risk of iron-deficiency anemia	Chia seeds, dark meat poultry, dates, green vegetables, lean beef, raisins, spinach	White Bean Chicken Chili (page 71), Chicken Sausage, Chickpea, and Kale Soup (page 72), Ginger Cashew Smoothie (page 34)

KEY NUTRIENT	BENEFITS	SUPERFOODS TO EAT	RECIPES
Magnesium	May help reduce leg cramps and may help support quality sleep	Arugula, avocados, chocolate, coconut water, flaxseed, legumes, milk, nuts, quinoa, tofu	Avocado, Almond, and Pear Salad (page 63), Tofu Breakfast Tacos with Avocado (page 28)
Vitamin A/ Beta Carotene	Helps support immune function and eye health	Carrots, mangos, red bell peppers	Lemon Artichoke Dip with Veggies (page 43), Orzo with Vegetables (page 59)
Vitamin B_6	May help offer nausea relief	Apples, bananas, broccoli, chicken, edamame, oats, peanut butter, pork, potatoes, popcorn	Oatmeal Cookies (page 109), Pita Chips with Edamame Hummus (page 40), Lemon-Thyme Pork Tenderloin (page 96)
Vitamin B_{12}	Supports healthy development of a baby's spinal cord; helps support energy levels and may help combat pregnancy fatigue	Chicken, eggs, lean beef, milk, salmon	Cheesy Beef Enchilada Casserole (page 88), Strip Steak with Caramelized Onions (page 93)
Vitamin C	Supports a healthy immune system and skin integrity	Blueberries, lemons, limes, strawberries, orange, tomatoes	Banana Berry Cashew Breakfast Bowl (page 24), Cheesecake-Stuffed Strawberries (page 104), Caprese Pasta Salad (page 62)
Vitamin D	Supports bone health and an overall healthy pregnancy	Milk, mushrooms, salmon, eggs	Quick Vegetarian "Beef" Lasagna (page 90), Tomato and Avocado Egg Scramble (page 29)
Zinc	Helps support immune function	Chicken, eggs, lean beef, milk, pistachios, walnuts, whole grains	Classic Chicken Noodle Soup (page 74), Grilled Chicken, Avocado, and Mango Salad (page 54)

Making Adjustments for Special Diets and Allergies

Eating for pregnancy doesn't have to be complicated. But there are occasions where making adjustments to meal plans and recipes are important depending on your individual dietary needs.

SPECIAL DIETS

There are many special diets out there these days, and while some can help us make healthier choices, they can leave a pregnant person with some nutritional gaps.

KETO: It is important to note that there is no data to suggest that following this way of eating is safe for a growing baby or for a pregnant person. For that reason alone, following a keto diet is not recommended during pregnancy.

PALEO: The paleo diet allows for a bit more variety in the macronutrient department, and therefore can be adjusted to be pregnancy safe as long as your health-care provider gives this diet the green light. Just make sure that you are filling in any potential nutrition gaps with proper supplementation. Calcium in particular can be challenging to get into a paleo diet in adequate amounts when dairy is avoided.

VEGAN: Many people follow a vegan lifestyle and give birth to healthy and happy babies. And while this way of eating can be a healthy choice for certain people, it does eliminate many foods that are rich in important pregnancy nutrients, like choline, vitamin B_{12}, and DHA omega-3 fatty acids. Again, supplementation may be necessary when following this diet. Ensuring that you are taking an algae-based DHA omega-3 supplement can help you meet your essential fatty acid needs without eating fish.

Food allergies affect many people, and when you are pregnant, the last thing you want to deal with is an allergic reaction.

Chances are, you are already aware of which foods you need to avoid if you are managing a food allergy. It is important to be mindful of which nutrients you may be missing out on when you avoid certain foods entirely, and to supplement accordingly. For example, if you are avoiding eggs, taking a choline supplement is a good idea. Avoiding seafood? DHA supplements may be necessary.

If you have any concerns about potential nutritional gaps due to your food allergy, especially when you are pregnant, consult with your health-care provider for personalized guidance.

Your Easy Pregnancy-Friendly Kitchen

Having a well-stocked kitchen makes it that much easier to prepare pregnancy-friendly meals. This book will rely on some staple ingredients and pieces of equipment, many of which you probably already have in your kitchen.

Although this list is not all-inclusive, here are some items I like to see in a pregnancy-friendly kitchen.

PANTRY AND COUNTER

- Bananas
- Black pepper
- Broth, chicken and vegetable
- Chickpeas, canned
- Cinnamon
- Crackers, whole grain
- Nut butter, natural
- Olive oil, extra-virgin
- Olives, canned
- Pasta, whole grain
- Pistachios, shelled
- Quinoa
- Salt
- Walnuts

GESTATIONAL DIABETES AND NUTRITION

When a person experiences gestational diabetes, their cells become resistant to insulin due to those pesky pregnancy hormones. In turn, the body has a hard time absorbing glucose, or sugar. While receiving a diagnosis of gestational diabetes can feel scary, the good news is that it is nothing that you can't manage with some dietary modifications and perhaps some medication, and many babies are born perfectly healthy to people who have this condition.

If you are managing gestational diabetes, here are some tips that may help you manage your blood sugar. Of course, it is always advisable to speak with a registered dietitian who can offer personalized advice and help you troubleshoot any challenges.

- Limit or avoid concentrated sweets like table sugar, cookies, cakes, and candies.

- Swap out sugary drinks like soda and sweet tea for water or sparkling water.

- Eat vegetables with most meals.

- Choose whole-grain carbs like whole-grain bread and quinoa instead of white bread and white rice.

- Keep on hand healthy and balanced snacks that contain some protein and healthy fats, like peanut butter crackers or a fruit and cheese plate.

- Include some physical activity in your day, as long as it is okay with your health-care provider.

In this book, recipes that are gestational diabetes–friendly are labeled "GDM-Friendly," so you know which dishes can be included in your diet. GDM-friendly recipes include Walnut-Crusted Salmon (page 92), Ginger Tofu Citrus Bowl (page 80), and Cinnamon Roasted Walnuts (page 42).

FIVE TIME-SAVING TIPS

Let's be real for a moment. When a person is pregnant, the last thing they want to do is chop, peel, and stay on their swollen feet standing over a hot stove. Here are some additional tips to make preparing and cooking meals easier.

1. **BATCH COOK:** If you just don't have much energy to cook during the week, pick a few of the recipes from this book to cook over the weekend, make double or triple batches, freeze them, and reheat what you need during the week.

2. **MEAL PLAN:** Taking an hour out of your week to plan meals can save you tons of time in the long run. Make a loose menu, draft a shopping list, and let your plan guide you for the entire week.

3. **BUY PRE-CHOPPED INGREDIENTS:** If your budget allows, buy onions, peppers, and other produce that are pre-chopped in order to save time in the kitchen.

4. **GET A PARTNER OR FRIEND INVOLVED:** Four hands can get the work done faster than two, so don't take the brunt of the labor onto your own shoulders. Solicit help from a partner, friend, or family member and get cooking!

5. **PLAN ON LEFTOVERS:** Use leftovers to your advantage. If you are eating grilled chicken breast for dinner, use the leftover chicken to top your salad at lunchtime. Get creative with whatever is left over so you can save time in the kitchen and minimize waste, too.

- Berries
- Carrots
- Chicken breast, frozen
- Citrus fruit
- Eggs
- Kale, spinach, or other dark leafy greens

- Lean beef, like flank steak or lean ground beef
- Milk, 2 percent
- Greek yogurt, plain
- Salmon
- Shrimp

EQUIPMENT ESSENTIALS

- Baking sheets
- Blender
- Cooking spatula
- Food processor

- Knives (sharp enough to cut through hard fruits and vegetables)
- Muffin tin
- Pots and pans

Sample Menus for Pesky Pregnancy Symptoms

In this section, you will find three sample weeklong menus for common pregnancy symptoms, using recipes from this book. Note that following these plans does not guarantee symptom relief, but they do maximize consumption of useful ingredients and help you stay away from foods that might exacerbate the condition. Because everyone's pregnancy is different, the sample menus don't mean that you *must* eat breakfast, lunch, dinner, and a snack every day. Customize these menus to suit your needs.

For nausea relief, spicy food and seafood should be limited. Ginger and carbohydrate-rich meals may support tolerance. Foods high in vitamin B_6 are also linked to improved nausea symptoms for some people.

If you can't stomach much food, it is important to make sure that, at the very least, you are getting enough fluids. Maintaining proper hydration is essential throughout your pregnancy. Sipping on broth or snacking on hydrating foods like watermelon and cucumber can help you keep your fluid balance in check.

DAY	BREAKFAST	LUNCH	DINNER	SNACK
MON	½ cup Greek yogurt with berries	Grilled cheese on whole-grain bread ½ banana Carrot sticks	Classic Chicken Noodle Soup (page 74) Sliced cucumbers and 2 kiwis	Whole-grain crackers and peanut butter
TUE	2 slices whole-grain toast topped with sliced avocado	*Leftover* Classic Chicken Noodle Soup	Ginger Tofu Citrus Bowl (page 80) 1 orange	Ginger Lemon Shot (page 100)
WED	Blueberry Banana Chia Smoothie (page 35)	*Leftover* Ginger Tofu Citrus Bowl	Lemony Ricotta Pasta with Crushed Pistachios (page 84)	Air-popped popcorn
THU	Protein-Boosting Oatmeal with Mixed Berries (Page 25)	*Leftover* Ricotta Pasta with Crushed Pistachios	Miso and Veggie Soup (page 75) Chicken and Quinoa Casserole with Broccoli (page 86)	1 cup fresh strawberries and a handful of nuts
FRI	Banana Berry Cashew Breakfast Bowl (page 24)	*Leftover* Miso and Veggie Soup Sliced pear and nut butter or cucumber slices	Chicken Piccata with Zoodles (page 94) Side salad (if desired)	Whole-grain crackers and sliced pasteurized cheese

SAT	Ginger Cashew Smoothie (page 34)	*Leftover* Chicken Piccata with Zoodles Side salad (if desired)	Chilled Ginger Carrot Soup (page 68) *Leftover* Chicken and Quinoa Casserole with Broccoli	Frozen Yogurt Blueberry Bites (page 47)
SUN	PB&J French Toast (page 27) 1 cup berries	*Leftover* Chilled Ginger Carrot Soup	Baked Potato Soup (page 76) Side salad (if desired)	Sliced apple and peanut butter

SWELLING AND PUFFINESS RELIEF

Ah, the joys of swollen ankles and puffy cheeks during pregnancy! While this is an all-too-common side effect of pregnancy, you can combat swelling and puffiness by watching your salt intake, eating plenty of veggies, and drinking lots of water.

DAY	BREAKFAST	LUNCH	DINNER	SNACK
MON	Sweet Greens Smoothie (page 36)	Kale with Chickpea Couscous (page 57) ½ cup berries	Grilled Chicken, Avocado, and Mango Salad (page 54) 1 slice wheat toast	Lemon Artichoke Dip with Veggies (page 43)
TUE	Zucchini Bread Oatmeal (page 32)	*Leftover* Grilled Chicken, Avocado, and Mango Salad	Chilled Ginger Carrot Soup (page 68) Whole-grain roll and 2 kiwis	Chocolate Cranberry Bark (page 106)
WED	Tomato and Avocado Egg Scramble (page 29)	*Leftover* Chilled Ginger Carrot Soup Whole-grain roll and ½ cup grapes	Walnut-Crusted Salmon (page 92) Cauliflower and Potato Mash (page 60)	Banana Kefir Shake (page 41)

THU	Protein-Boosting Oatmeal with Mixed Berries (page 25)	*Leftover* Walnut-Crusted Salmon *Leftover* Cauliflower Mash	Ginger Tofu Citrus Bowl (page 80)	1 cup fresh berries and string cheese
FRI	Banana Berry Cashew Breakfast Bowl (page 24)	*Leftover* Ginger Tofu Citrus Bowl	Salmon Salad with Dates (page 55) 2 mandarin oranges	1 frozen yogurt bar (store-bought)
SAT	Ginger Cashew Smoothie (page 34)	*Leftover* Salmon Salad with Dates	Vegan Buddha Bowl (page 85) 1 cup cubed melon	Sliced carrots and cucumbers with hummus
SUN	Papaya Chia Pudding (page 31)	*Leftover* Vegan Buddha Bowl	Strip Steak with Caramelized Onions (page 93) with side salad (if desired) Cheesecake-Stuffed Strawberries (page 104)	4 pitted dates stuffed with almond butter

FIVE SNACKS TO PACK IN YOUR GO BAG

If you haven't already heard, hospital food can be lackluster, to put it mildly. And, depending on what time you give birth, the hospital kitchen may not even be open. So, packing some nutrient-rich snacks in your hospital bag is a wise move. If you don't end up eating the items you packed, share them with your kind nurses.

Here are some yummy and perfectly portable snacks you can pack in your hospital go bag (even weeks before it's go time):

- Dried fruit with no added sugar or sulfur dioxide (some great choices include mangos, raisins, and apples)

- Mixed nuts

- Cinnamon Roasted Walnuts (page 42)

- Low-sugar granola bars

ENERGY BOOST

While there is no magic bullet to help you feel a little more energized, eating nutrient-rich foods with complex carbs can give you a little zing when you need it.

DAY	BREAKFAST	LUNCH	DINNER	SNACK
MON	Zucchini Bread Oatmeal (page 32)	Grilled Chicken, Avocado, and Mango Salad (page 54) Slice of whole-grain toast	Mexican-Inspired Baked Potatoes (page 82) 1 orange	Chicory Coffee Latte (page 48)
TUE	Papaya Chia Pudding (page 31)	*Leftover* Mexican Baked Potato	Vegan Buddha Bowl (page 85) 1 cup watermelon	Banana Kefir Shake (page 41)

WED	Tofu Breakfast Tacos with Avocado (page 28)	*Leftover* Vegan Buddha Bowl	Quick Vegetarian "Beef" Lasagna (page 90) Side salad	1 orange and string cheese
THU	PB&J French Toast (page 27)	*Leftover* Quick Vegetarian "Beef" Lasagna Side salad	Cheesy Beef Enchilada Casserole (page 88) 2 kiwis	Pita Chips with Edamame Hummus (page 40)
FRI	Coconut Melon Smoothie (page 33)	*Leftover* Cheesy Beef Enchilada Casserole	Caprese Pasta Salad (page 62)	Carrot sticks with natural peanut butter
SAT	Breakfast Parfait with Tahini, Maple Syrup, and Figs (page 26)	*Leftover* Caprese Pasta Salad	Lentil Carrot Soup (page 70) 6 whole-grain crackers	½ cup walnuts and 1 ounce dark chocolate
SUN	*Leftover* Breakfast Parfait with Tahini, Maple Syrup, and Figs	*Leftover* Lentil Carrot Soup	Tex-Mex Naan Pizzas (page 83) Sliced tomato and avocado	Date Energy Balls (page 45)

About the Recipes

The main focus of this book is on simplicity. Each recipe has seven or fewer main ingredients (excluding water, salt, pepper, and oil or cooking spray. With some recipes, you'll also see ingredients that are labeled as optional. I've included them because a squeeze of lime may add brightness to a dish, or a pinch of red pepper flakes a little heat. But they are not needed for flavor or nutritional value, and you should feel free to skip over them if you choose. To help make preparation easier, many of the recipes fall into one of three categories of ease, indicated by the following labels: Quick, One-Pot, and Freezer-Friendly.

The dishes include only ingredients that have been shown to be safe for pregnancy, and they exclude any items that are even remotely questionable. In addition, I've made sure to include superfoods in every recipe to ensure you and your baby are getting key nutrients.

All recipes have labels that will help you quicky reference specific aspects of your pregnancy experience you want or need to address. You can also refer to the Symptom Index (page 124) to search for recipes by symptom labels. These labels include:

- CONSTIPATION AID

- ENERGY BOOSTER

- GESTATIONAL DIABETES—FRIENDLY (GDM-FRIENDLY)

- LACTATION SUPPORT

- NAUSEA RELIEF

- POSTPARTUM RECOVERY

- SWELLING RELIEF

Pregnancy can be challenging—but feeding yourself should be enjoyable and easy. I can't wait to show you how delicious and simple it can be to nourish your body and baby during this time. Let's get started!

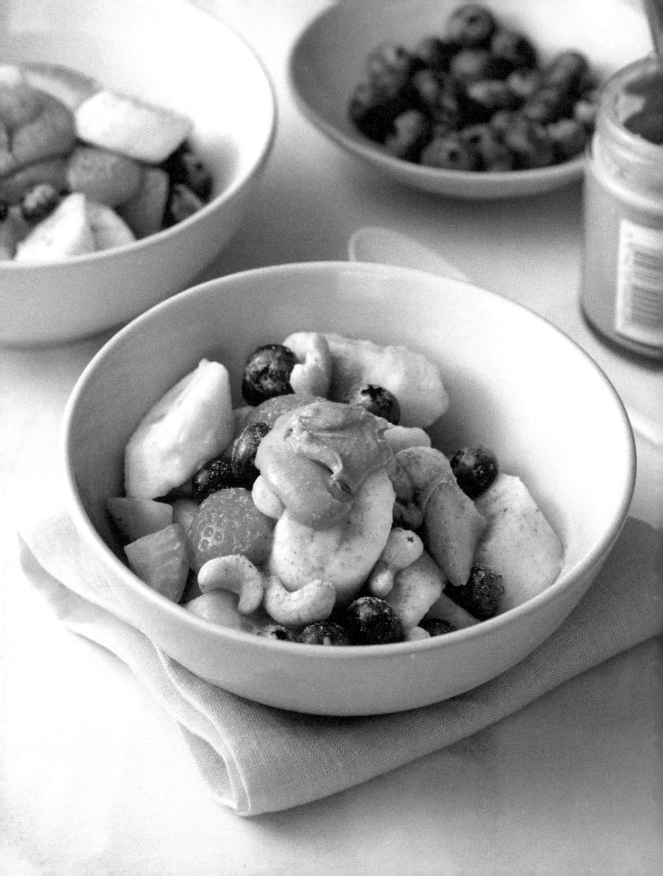

TWO

BREAKFAST AND SMOOTHIES

< BANANA BERRY CASHEW
BREAKFAST BOWL (PAGE 24)

BANANA BERRY CASHEW BREAKFAST BOWL

Serves 4 • Prep time: 5 MINUTES

GDM-Friendly | Lactation Support | Nausea Relief | Quick

This simple breakfast can be put together in no time. While it is intentionally on the bland side to soothe nausea, feel free to jazz it up with some cinnamon or other spices if your stomach can handle it.

4 bananas, peeled

1 cup cashews

½ cup blueberries

½ cup strawberries, quartered

¼ cup unsalted cashew butter

½ teaspoon ground ginger

1. Slice the bananas into ½-inch pieces.

2. Put the bananas, cashews, blueberries, and strawberries in a bowl. Gently toss to combine.

3. Divide the fruit-and-nut mixture among 4 serving bowls. Drizzle with cashew butter and top with ginger.

SUBSTITUTION TIP: Feel free to swap in your favorite fruit or nut butter to your taste.

Per serving (1 cup): Calories: 396; Total fat: 23g; Saturated fat: 4g; Carbohydrates: 46g; Sugar: 20g; Fiber: 5g; Protein: 10g

PROTEIN-BOOSTING OATMEAL WITH MIXED BERRIES

Serves 4 • **Prep time:** 5 MINUTES • **Cook time:** 10 MINUTES

Lactation Support | Nausea Relief | One-Pot | Quick | Swelling Relief

Protein needs increase as your pregnancy progresses. Starting your day with protein-packed oatmeal can help you feel satisfied until lunchtime. Adding collagen peptides to your oatmeal is a simple way to sneak some pregnancy-fueling amino acids into your diet.

2 cups rolled oats

3 cups 2 percent milk

2 medium bananas, mashed

1½ teaspoons vanilla extract

1 teaspoon ground cinnamon

Pinch salt

3 tablespoons unflavored collagen peptides

1 cup berries of choice, washed

1. In a small saucepan over medium-high heat, combine the oats, milk, bananas, vanilla, cinnamon, and salt and bring to a boil.

2. Reduce the heat to medium-low and cook for 5 minutes, stirring occasionally.

3. Remove the saucepan from the heat and stir in the collagen peptides.

4. Divide the oatmeal among 4 bowls. Top with berries before serving.

MAKE IT EASIER: Leftovers can be kept covered in the refrigerator for up to 3 days. Reheat in the microwave for 1 minute or on the stove in a small pot.

Per serving (1 cup cooked oats with toppings): Calories: 347; Total fat: 7g; Saturated fat: 3g; Carbohydrates: 56g; Sugar: 21g; Fiber: 7g; Protein: 18g

BREAKFAST PARFAIT WITH TAHINI, MAPLE SYRUP, AND FIGS

Serves 4 • Prep time: 5 MINUTES • Cook time: 20 SECONDS

Energy Booster | Postpartum Recovery | Quick

Breakfast parfaits look fancy, but they are one of the simplest things you can whip up. Starting your day with Greek yogurt fuels the body with high-quality protein and the natural calcium supports bone health.

½ cup tahini

¼ cup pure maple syrup

2 cups 2 percent vanilla Greek yogurt, divided

4 fresh figs, thinly sliced

½ cup slivered almonds

1. In a small bowl, combine the tahini and maple syrup and microwave on high for 20 seconds. Remove the mixture from the microwave and stir until well combined. Set aside to cool.

2. Take out 4 serving bowls or mason jars. Put 2 tablespoons of yogurt into each bowl.

3. Layer the figs on top of the yogurt in each bowl.

4. Once the tahini and syrup has cooled, drizzle 1 tablespoon per serving over the figs.

5. Evenly divide the remaining 1½ cups of yogurt among the 4 bowls (about 6 tablespoons each).

6. Sprinkle 2 tablespoons of almonds over each serving.

7. Drizzle an equal portion of the remaining tahini-maple syrup sauce over each serving.

SUBSTITUTION TIP: Swap out the Greek yogurt with a nondairy yogurt for a vegan-friendly breakfast.

MAKE IT EASIER: Make this in a mason jar the night before and leave it in your refrigerator with the lid on for a quick grab-and-go breakfast.

Per serving (½ cup yogurt with toppings): Calories: 467; Total fat: 26g; Saturated fat: 4g; Carbohydrates: 45g; Sugar: 35g; Fiber: 6g; Protein: 18g

PB&J FRENCH TOAST

Serves 4 • Prep time: 5 MINUTES • Cook time: 15 MINUTES

Constipation Relief | Nausea Relief | Quick

What is better than a classic PB&J? Why, PB&J French toast, of course! Packed with protein and goodness, this easy breakfast will surely satisfy, even if you don't feel like you can stomach a thing. This calls for fruit jam instead of jelly, but if you are really craving the old-school grape jelly, go for it, since the chia seeds sneak in some added fiber.

8 slices whole-grain bread

½ cup unsalted natural peanut butter

4 tablespoons fruit jam

1 tablespoon chia seeds

4 tablespoons unsalted butter, divided

2 eggs

½ cup 2 percent milk

1. Lay out 4 slices of bread. Spread 2 tablespoons of the peanut butter on top of each slice.

2. Spread 1 tablespoon of jam on top of the peanut butter and sprinkle an equal portion of chia seeds over the jam on each slice of bread. Place the remaining 4 slices of bread on top of the peanut butter and jam to make a sandwich.

3. In a large skillet or frying pan, melt 1 tablespoon of butter over medium heat.

4. Meanwhile, in a medium bowl, whisk together the eggs and milk. Dip 1 sandwich into the egg and milk mixture until fully coated.

5. Transfer the coated sandwich to the skillet (you should be able to fit 2 sandwiches in a large skillet at a time) and cook for 3 minutes on each side. Transfer the cooked sandwiches to a plate.

6. Repeat steps 4 and 5 with the remaining 2 sandwiches.

MAKE IT EASIER: Whip up your basic sandwiches the night before, then batter and cook them in the morning.

Per serving (1 sandwich): Calories: 612; Total fat: 35g; Saturated fat: 12g; Carbohydrates: 55g; Sugar: 17g; Fiber: 10g; Protein: 23g

TOFU BREAKFAST TACOS WITH AVOCADO

Makes 8 tacos • Prep time: 15 MINUTES • Cook time: 15 MINUTES

Energy Booster | GDM-Friendly | Lactation Support | Postpartum Recovery | Quick

Tacos for breakfast? Absolutely! Enjoying tofu tacos in the morning gives your body a boost of protein and tons of baby-friendly nutrients. To include even more baby-friendly nutrients in this dish, feel free to add a scrambled egg.

10 ounces firm tofu

1 cup canned black beans

1 tablespoon extra-virgin olive oil

1 teaspoon garlic powder

½ teaspoon chili powder

1 teaspoon salt

8 whole-grain corn tortillas

2 ripe avocados, peeled and sliced

1 cup store-bought salsa

1 bunch cilantro, chopped (optional)

½ lime, sliced (optional)

1. Wrap the tofu in paper towels and place something heavy on top, such as a textbook or cast-iron skillet. Set aside.

2. In a medium saucepan over medium heat, cook the black beans with their liquid for 5 minutes, then remove the pan from the heat.

3. In a large skillet, heat the oil over medium heat for about 2 minutes, or until sizzling.

4. Meanwhile, unwrap the tofu and use a butter knife to crumble it.

5. Once the oil is sizzling, put the crumbled tofu along with the garlic, chili powder, and salt into the skillet and cook for 4 to 5 minutes, or until browned.

6. Wrap the tortillas with paper towels sprinkled with water and heat in the microwave on high for 10 seconds.

7. Top the warm tortillas with the tofu scramble, warmed black beans, avocado slices, salsa, cilantro, and a squeeze of lime (if using).

SUBSTITUTION TIP: For a milder version of this taco, skip the chili powder and cumin.

Per serving (2 tacos): Calories: 397; Total fat: 19g; Saturated fat: 3g; Carbohydrates: 45g; Sugar: 4g; Fiber: 14g; Protein: 15g

TOMATO AND AVOCADO EGG SCRAMBLE

Serves 4 • Prep time: 5 MINUTES • Cook time: 8 MINUTES

GDM-Friendly | Lactation Support | One-Pot | Swelling Relief

An egg scramble is a busy person's dream come true. Toss everything in a pan, cook, and enjoy! Plus, eating eggs during pregnancy is one of the best things you can do for your little one's developing brain.

4 slices natural turkey bacon

2 cups cherry tomatoes

8 eggs

2 tablespoons 2 percent milk

½ teaspoon salt

1 ripe avocado, sliced

1. Heat a large skillet over medium heat. Cook the bacon until crispy, about 3 minutes on each side. Transfer the bacon to a plate and set aside.

2. Without cleaning out the skillet, add the tomatoes and cook them for 4 minutes, or until soft.

3. Break apart the bacon and sprinkle the pieces over the tomatoes.

4. In a large bowl, whisk together the eggs, milk, and salt. Pour the egg mixture into the skillet and stir gently for 5 minutes, or until the scrambled eggs are cooked through and no longer runny.

5. Serve with avocado slices.

SUBSTITUTION TIP: Make this a complete breakfast by serving with a slice of whole-grain toast and a glass of 100 percent pure orange juice. For some extra flavor, top the eggs with a dollop of pasteurized goat cheese.

Per serving (½ cup): Calories: 242; Total fat: 16g; Saturated fat: 4g; Carbohydrates: 7g; Sugar: 3g; Fiber: 3g; Protein: 18g

CHICKEN SAUSAGE QUICHE

Serves 6 • Prep time: 5 MINUTES • Cook time: 40 MINUTES

Freezer-Friendly | Lactation Support

Quiche is an easy dish that can be enjoyed for any meal of the day. The addition of chicken gives this dish important pregnancy nutrients like choline and vitamin B_{12}. Using panko bread crumbs instead of a classic crust saves this dish a significant amount of empty calories while still giving it a satisfying taste.

Cooking spray

2½ tablespoons panko bread crumbs

½ pound natural chicken sausage

½ cup onion, chopped

½ cup button mushrooms, chopped

4 ounces fresh broccoli, chopped

6 eggs

1 cup whole milk

Salt

Freshly ground black pepper

Parmesan cheese, for garnish (optional)

1. Preheat the oven to 425°F. Spray a 9½-inch pie plate with cooking spray. Spread the bread crumbs evenly on the pie plate.

2. In a medium saucepan over medium-high heat, cook the sausage for 5 to 7 minutes, until lightly browned. Remove the meat from the pan and drain the fat.

3. Lower the heat to medium and reheat the pan. Combine the onion, mushrooms, and broccoli and sauté for 5 minutes. Remove the pan from the heat.

4. In a medium bowl, whisk together the eggs and milk until combined.

5. Place the cooked sausage and vegetables evenly into prepared pie plate. Pour the eggs on top. Sprinkle with Parmesan cheese (if using) and bake for 25 minutes or until the eggs are cooked through.

MAKE IT EASIER: To freeze, let this dish cool completely, cover, and freeze for up to 2 months. To enjoy again, let the quiche thaw completely in the refrigerator before cooking at 425°F for 25 minutes.

Per serving (1 slice): Calories: 182; Total fat: 10g; Saturated fat: 3g; Carbohydrates: 9g; Sugar: 4g; Fiber: 1g; Protein: 14g

PAPAYA CHIA PUDDING

Serves 4 • Prep time: 5 MINUTES, PLUS 7 HOURS OR OVERNIGHT TO SET

Constipation Aid | Energy Booster | Postpartum Recovery | Swelling Relief

Chia pudding is the secret weapon for anyone dealing with constipation. Packed with both soluble and insoluble fiber, these little seeds pack a nutritional punch. Sweetening this pudding with fruit instead of sugar gives your body additional beneficial vitamins and minerals. You can also make one large batch of the pudding and divide it into individual portions after it sets in the refrigerator.

1 ripe papaya, peeled and halved, seeded

1 cup chia seeds

1 teaspoon ground cinnamon

2 cups coconut milk

1 tablespoon crushed macadamia nuts

1½ teaspoons coconut flakes

1. Put the papaya in a medium bowl. Using a fork or a potato masher, mash the papaya.

2. In a separate bowl, whisk together the chia seeds, cinnamon, and coconut milk.

3. Divide the papaya among 4 glass bowls or mason jars to make up the bottom layer. Then divide the chia mixture evenly among the bowls.

4. Cover and let sit in the refrigerator for 1 hour. Remove the covers, stir, and cover again. Leave in refrigerator for at least 6 hours more or overnight.

5. When you are ready to eat, sprinkle an equal portion of macadamia nuts and coconut flakes over each serving.

SUBSTITUTION TIP: If you can't find papaya, use a peeled and pitted mango or 2 peaches instead.

Per serving (½ cup chia pudding with toppings): Calories: 494; Total fat: 39g; Saturated fat: 19g; Carbohydrates: 35g; Sugar: 11g; Fiber: 15g; Protein: 10g

ZUCCHINI BREAD OATMEAL

Serves 4 • Prep time: 5 MINUTES • Cook time: 10 MINUTES

Constipation Aid | Energy Booster | Lactation Support | Nausea Relief
One-Pot | Postpartum Recovery | Quick | Swelling Relief

When you are feeling queasy or sluggish, eating vegetables may be the last thing on your mind. This nourishing oatmeal is packed with nutritious ingredients like zucchini and walnuts to help keep you going. Plus, the natural fiber found in most of these ingredients will help keep constipation at bay.

2 zucchini

3 cups 2 percent milk, or milk of choice

2 cups rolled oats

½ teaspoon salt

2 teaspoons ground cinnamon

¼ cup pure maple syrup

2 teaspoons vanilla extract

¼ cup chopped walnuts

1. Grate the zucchini on the large holes of a box grater or chop it into small pieces.

2. In a medium saucepan, bring the milk to a boil over medium-high heat.

3. Stir in the oats and salt and cook for 2 minutes.

4. Reduce the heat to low. When the oatmeal starts to simmer, stir in the grated zucchini, cinnamon, maple syrup, and vanilla. Cook for 7 minutes more, or until most of the liquid is absorbed.

5. Divide among 4 serving bowls and top with walnuts before serving.

SUBSTITUTION TIP: For even more protein, add a scoop of unflavored protein powder to the oatmeal mixture after the oats complete their simmer at the end of step 4.

Per serving (1 cup oatmeal with walnuts): Calories: 370; Total fat: 11g; Saturated fat: 3g; Carbohydrates: 55g; Sugar: 25g; Fiber: 6g; Protein: 14g

COCONUT MELON SMOOTHIE

Serves 1 • Prep time: 5 MINUTES

Energy Booster | Nausea Relief | Postpartum Recovery | Quick | Swelling Relief

Sipping on a smoothie is an effortless way to get some nutrition. And this one, loaded with key nutrients like potassium, calcium, and folate, is hydrating, nourishing, and full of oh-so-good flavors. It's a great pick-me-up on days when you might not be feeling your best, or when you need a great thirst quencher.

1 cup honeydew melon chunks

½ frozen banana

1 cup coconut water

1 cup 2 percent plain Greek yogurt

¼ teaspoon ground nutmeg

¼ cup spinach

¼ cup ice

In a blender, combine the melon, banana, coconut water, yogurt, nutmeg, spinach, and ice and blend until smooth.

SUBSTITUTION TIP: On a hot day, skip the yogurt and add more ice for increased hydration.

Per serving (about 1 cup): Calories: 346; Total fat: 6g; Saturated fat: 3g; Carbohydrates: 48g; Sugar: 38g; Fiber: 3g; Protein: 26g

GINGER CASHEW SMOOTHIE

Serves 1 • Prep time: 5 MINUTES

Energy Booster | Nausea Relief | Postpartum Recovery | Quick | Swelling Relief

If nausea has struck, sipping on this smoothie may offer some relief, thanks to the fresh ginger. In addition, both bananas and milk naturally contain vitamin B_6, a nutrient that is linked to nausea support.

1 cup 2 percent milk

2 teaspoons minced fresh ginger

¼ teaspoon ground cinnamon

¼ teaspoon ground nutmeg

½ frozen banana

2 pitted Medjool dates

1 tablespoon unsalted cashew butter

½ cup ice

In a blender, combine the milk, ginger, cinnamon, nutmeg, banana, dates, cashew butter, and ice and blend until smooth.

SUBSTITUTION TIP: Swap out the 2 percent milk for a nondairy alternative if it is easier on your system, or if you prefer a vegan smoothie.

Per serving (about 1 cup): Calories: 415; Total fat: 13g; Saturated fat: 5g; Carbohydrates: 69g; Sugar: 53g; Fiber: 6g; Protein: 13g

BLUEBERRY BANANA CHIA SMOOTHIE

Serves 1 • Prep time: 5 MINUTES

Constipation Aid | Energy Booster | Freezer-Friendly | GDM-Friendly
Lactation Support | Nausea Relief | Postpartum Recovery | Quick | Swelling Relief

If you are trying to manage constipation in a natural way, this smoothie is for you. The addition of the blueberries provides an antioxidant boost that helps keep you healthy during pregnancy. Using fermented kefir instead of milk gives this smoothie some live probiotics, which may help keep your bowel movements regular.

1 tablespoon chia seeds

1 tablespoon unsalted almond butter

½ banana

1 cup unsweetened kefir

⅔ cup frozen blueberries

3 pitted Medjool dates

½ cup ice

In a blender, combine the chia seeds, almond butter, banana, kefir, blueberries, dates, and ice and blend until smooth.

MAKE IT EASIER: Freeze leftover smoothies in ice pop molds for a cool and nutritious treat.

Per serving (about 1 cup): Calories: 635; Total fat: 22g; Saturated fat: 6g; Carbohydrates: 106g; Sugar: 81g; Fiber: 15g; Protein: 16g

SWEET GREENS SMOOTHIE

Serves 1 • Prep time: 5 MINUTES
Energy Booster | Lactation Support | Nausea Relief
Postpartum Recovery | Quick | Swelling Relief

Eating dark leafy greens is one of the best things you can do for yourself and for your baby, but sometimes a salad during pregnancy is simply unappealing. The answer is a green smoothie—a blend of greens, fruit, and protein that gives you a balanced nutritional boost. Think of it like a salad in a glass.

2 kiwis, peeled and cubed

½ frozen banana

½ cup spinach

½ cup kale

½ cup milk of choice

½ cup 2 percent vanilla Greek yogurt

1 scoop unflavored collagen peptides

In a blender, combine the kiwis, banana, spinach, kale, milk, yogurt, and collagen peptides and blend until smooth.

SUBSTITUTION TIP: Feel free to use any leafy green veggie you have on hand if you don't have kale or spinach. Even frozen chopped cauliflower will work well in this smoothie.

Per serving (about 1 cup): Calories: 295; Total fat: 3g; Saturated fat: 2g; Carbohydrates: 47g; Sugar: 32g; Fiber: 6g; Protein: 23g

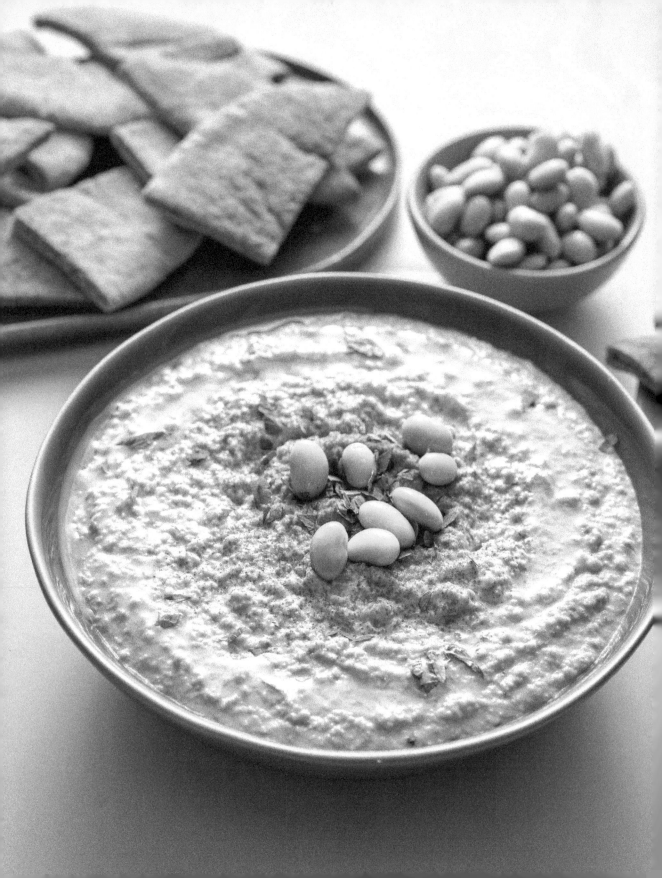

THREE

SNACKS

< PITA CHIPS WITH EDAMAME
HUMMUS (PAGE 40)

PITA CHIPS WITH EDAMAME HUMMUS

Serves 6 • **Prep time:** 10 MINUTES • **Cook time:** 15 MINUTES
Energy Booster | GDM-Friendly | Quick | Swelling Relief

Some of the most satisfying snacks involve crunching and dipping, and this recipe gives you both. Loaded with whole grains, plant-based protein, and fiber, this snack is delicious, easy to make, and will help keep you going on a busy day.

3 (6-inch) whole-grain pitas, halved

1 cup frozen unsalted shelled edamame, thawed

1 tablespoon extra-virgin olive oil

¼ teaspoon salt

1 garlic clove, peeled

2 tablespoons tahini

2 tablespoons water

1 tablespoon freshly squeezed lemon juice

¼ teaspoon ground cumin

1. Preheat the oven to 365°F.

2. Place the pita halves in a single layer directly on the oven rack and bake for 15 minutes, or until crispy—but not burnt.

3. Remove the baked pitas from the oven, let them cool, and then break them into pieces.

4. In a food processor, combine the edamame, oil, salt, garlic, tahini, water, lemon juice, and cumin and process to form a smooth paste.

5. Transfer the edamame mixture to a bowl and serve with pita crackers for dipping.

SUBSTITUTION TIP: You can add extra garlic or additional spices, like paprika, parsley, and coriander, to your taste and tolerance level.

Per serving (½ pita and 2 tablespoons hummus): Calories: 157; Total fat: 7g; Saturated fat: 1g; Carbohydrates: 20g; Sugar: 2g; Fiber: 3g; Protein: 6g

BANANA KEFIR SHAKE

Serves 1 • **Prep time:** 5 MINUTES

Constipation Aid | Energy Booster | Nausea Relief

Postpartum Recovery | Quick | Swelling Relief

Similar to yogurt, kefir is packed with live probiotics, or live bacteria, that can help keep your gut healthy and offer some constipation relief. This "shake" has far fewer calories than traditional milkshakes with far more nutrients to boot. The banana and date add some natural sweetness and nutrients without any added sugars!

1 cup vanilla kefir

1 banana

¼ teaspoon ground cinnamon

1 pitted Medjool date

In a blender, combine the kefir, banana, cinnamon, and date and blend until smooth.

SUBSTITUTION TIP: Use a frozen banana for a thicker shake. If you can tolerate spice, try swapping out the cinnamon for a dash of cayenne pepper.

Per serving: (1 cup) Calories: 373; Total fat: 9g; Saturated fat: 6g; Carbohydrates: 65g; Sugar: 45g; Fiber: 6g; Protein: 12g

CINNAMON ROASTED WALNUTS

Makes 4 cups • Prep time: 10 MINUTES • Cook time: 20 MINUTES
Constipation Aid | Energy Booster | Freezer-Friendly | GDM-Friendly
Lactation Support | Nausea Relief | Postpartum Recovery | Quick | Swelling Relief

Walnuts are a nutritional powerhouse and make an awesome grab-and-go snack. The addition of warming cinnamon makes walnuts even tastier. Along with awesome flavor, you will be getting healthy fats, fiber, and plant-based protein to keep you fueled and satisfied.

Cooking spray

1 egg white

1 tablespoon water

4 cups walnut halves

¼ cup brown sugar

1 tablespoon ground cinnamon

1 teaspoon salt

½ teaspoon ground nutmeg

½ teaspoon ground ginger

1. Preheat the oven to 350°F. Lightly coat the surface of a baking sheet with cooking spray.

2. In a large bowl, whisk together the egg white and water. Add the walnuts and toss to coat, covering each nut with the egg wash.

3. In a small bowl, whisk together the brown sugar, cinnamon, salt, nutmeg, and ginger. Sprinkle the spice mix over the coated nuts and toss to combine.

4. Spread the spiced nuts in a single layer on the prepared baking sheet and bake for 15 minutes, or until golden brown.

5. Stir and cook for 3 minutes more. Remove from the oven and let cool before serving.

6. Store in an airtight container in the refrigerator for up to 1 month, or in the freezer for up to 6 months.

SUBSTITUTION TIP: To try something different, you can swap out the walnuts for almonds.

Per serving (¼ cup): Calories: 175; Total fat: 16g; Saturated fat: 2g; Carbohydrates: 6g; Sugar: 3g; Fiber: 2g; Protein: 4g

LEMON ARTICHOKE DIP WITH VEGGIES

Serves 4 to 6 • Prep time: 5 MINUTES

GDM-Friendly | Lactation Support | Quick | Swelling Relief

Double your dose of vegetables with this quick and delicious dip. Packed with nutrient-dense superfoods like carrots and olive oil, this dish is a tasty way to add more fiber to your diet. To keep the sodium level of this snack low and to help with swelling, make sure you drain the artichoke hearts to remove as much salt as possible.

1¾ cups jarred artichoke hearts, drained

Juice of ½ lemon

¼ cup extra-virgin olive oil

2 tablespoons chopped fresh parsley

1 tablespoon minced garlic

4 ounces baby carrots

1 red bell pepper, sliced

1. In a food processor, combine the artichoke hearts, lemon juice, oil, parsley, and garlic. Process until smooth.

2. Transfer the mixture to a dipping bowl. Serve with carrots and red bell pepper slices.

MAKE IT EASIER: Use the leftover dip as a zingy condiment on a turkey sandwich.

Per serving (1 tablespoon dip plus vegetables): Calories: 173; Total fat: 14g; Saturated fat: 2g; Carbohydrates: 14g; Sugar: 3g; Fiber: 9g; Protein: 3g

PICKLE POPCORN

Serves 4 • Prep time: 5 MINUTES

Constipation Aid | Energy Booster | GDM-Friendly | Postpartum Recovery | Quick

Pickles, a famous pregnancy food, can certainly satisfy. While those crunchy and salty delights can be part of a healthy pregnancy diet, they aren't very filling and don't offer much nutrition. This popcorn is packed with pickle flavor, but also provides extra whole grains for sustained energy and some fiber to help combat constipation.

¼ teaspoon dillweed

⅛ teaspoon salt

⅛ teaspoon garlic powder

⅛ teaspoon ground coriander

½ tablespoon pickle juice

4 cups air-popped popcorn

1. In a small bowl, combine the dillweed, salt, garlic powder, coriander, and pickle juice.

2. Pour the popcorn into a large serving bowl.

3. Drizzle the spice mixture on top of the popcorn and toss to combine.

MAKE IT EASIER: Store this popcorn in smaller bags for a quick grab-and-go snack when your pickle craving hits.

Per serving (1 cup): Calories: 32; Total fat: <1g; Saturated fat: <1g; Carbohydrates: 6g; Sugar: <1g; Fiber: 1g; Protein: 1g

DATE ENERGY BALLS

Makes 12 energy balls • Prep time: 5 MINUTES, PLUS 1 HOUR TO CHILL

Constipation Aid | Energy Booster | Freezer-Friendly | Lactation Support

Dates are one of the best things that you can eat during pregnancy. Studies suggest that eating these little fruits during the last month of pregnancy can help make labor and delivery a little easier. These energy balls are the ultimate snack for busy days or for afternoons when you need a healthy pick-me-up.

½ cup pitted Medjool dates

2 tablespoons unsalted almond butter

½ cup rolled oats

Pinch salt

1½ teaspoons chia seeds

1 tablespoon dark chocolate chips

1. Line a baking sheet with parchment paper.

2. Put the dates into a food processor and process until the dates are in small pieces.

3. Add in the almond butter, oats, salt, and chia seeds and process until smooth.

4. Transfer the date and almond butter mixture to a medium bowl. Add the chocolate chips and mix until combined.

5. Using damp hands, roll the mixture into 12 (1-inch) balls.

6. Place the balls on the prepared baking sheet, and chill in the refrigerator for at least 1 hour before serving.

7. Leftovers can be stored in an airtight container in the refrigerator for up to 3 days.

MAKE IT EASIER: Make a double or triple recipe of energy balls and store them in an airtight container in the freezer for up to 3 months. Thaw enough for 2 or 3 portions at a time in refrigerator as needed.

Per serving (3 energy balls): Calories: 197; Total fat: 7g; Saturated fat: 1g; Carbohydrates: 34g; Sugar: 22g; Fiber: 5g; Protein: 4g

RANCH ZUCCHINI CHIPS

Serves 2 • Prep time: 10 MINUTES **• Cook time:** 1 HOUR 30 MINUTES

Constipation Aid | Energy Booster

These healthy zucchini chips will be your new go-to pregnancy snack when you're craving the crunch of those irresistible Cool Ranch Doritos. I love zucchini for their vitamin B, fiber, and mineral content. You can make this snack even if you don't have all the spices listed. A little garlic powder and salt can be quite satisfying.

2 zucchini, thinly cut into coins

2 teaspoons garlic powder

2 teaspoons onion powder

1 teaspoon dried oregano

1 teaspoon dried parsley

1 teaspoon dried dill

½ teaspoon dried chives

½ teaspoon salt

Freshly ground black pepper

1 tablespoon extra-virgin olive oil

1. Preheat the oven to 225°F. Line a baking pan with parchment paper.

2. Pat the zucchini coins with paper towels to draw out excess moisture.

3. In a small bowl, mix the garlic powder, onion powder, oregano, parsley, dill, chives, salt, and pepper.

4. In a large bowl, toss the zucchini with the oil. Sprinkle in the seasonings, making sure to coat each piece as evenly as possible.

5. Arrange the coins in a single layer on the baking sheet. Bake for 90 minutes, until completely dried out and crispy, checking at the 1-hour mark. Let cool to room temperature before serving.

Make It Easier: Use a mandoline, if you have one, to get the zucchini coins extra thin. The thinner the slices, the faster they'll cook.

Per serving: Calories: 115; Total fat: 8g; Saturated fat: 1g; Carbohydrates: 11g; Sugar: 5g; Fiber: 3g; Protein: 3g

FROZEN YOGURT BLUEBERRY BITES

Serves 4 • Prep time: 5 MINUTES • Total time: 55 MINUTES

Constipation Aid | Energy Booster | Freezer-Friendly | GDM-Friendly
Lactation Support | Nausea Relief | Postpartum Recovery | Swelling Relief

Blueberries are a nutritional powerhouse, full of antioxidants, fiber, and vitamin C. And while they are delicious on their own, sometimes they need a little more oomph. Coating fresh blueberries with Greek yogurt and then freezing them gives you a delightful snack with a tasty boost of protein, carbohydrates, fiber, and live probiotics.

2 cups blueberries, washed and dried

2 cups 2 percent plain Greek yogurt

1. Line a baking sheet with parchment paper.

2. Using a toothpick, dip each blueberry in yogurt and place the yogurt-covered berry on a baking sheet. Repeat with the remaining berries, arranging them on the sheet without touching one another.

3. Place the baking sheet in the freezer for 50 to 55 minutes, or until completely frozen.

4. Store the berries in a zip-top freezer bag in the freezer for up to 3 months.

SUBSTITUTION TIP: Swap out the blueberries for raspberries or blackberries.

Per serving (½ cup): Calories: 129; Total fat: 3g; Saturated fat: 2g; Carbohydrates: 14g; Sugar: 11g; Fiber: 2g; Protein: 13g

CHICORY COFFEE LATTE

Serves 4 • Cook time: 5 MINUTES

GDM-Friendly | Postpartum Recovery | Quick

If you are avoiding coffee but crave the ritual of the morning brew, this pregnancy-safe, caffeine-free chicory coffee latte can fill the void. You can enjoy the chicory coffee on its own, but this latte version provides extra protein and micronutrients like manganese that both you and your baby can benefit from.

2 tablespoons chicory root "coffee" grounds

2 cups boiling water

2 cups 2 percent milk

1 tablespoon pure maple syrup

1 teaspoon ground cinnamon

1. In a small saucepan, steep the chicory root grounds in boiling water for 5 minutes.

2. Meanwhile, in a separate small saucepan, combine the milk, maple syrup, and cinnamon. Warm over medium-low heat for 5 minutes, stirring to avoid burning the bottom of the pan.

3. Strain the chicory root coffee into the milk mixture and stir to combine.

4. Divide into 4 coffee mugs and serve immediately.

SUBSTITUTION TIP: Instead of cinnamon, add a dash of cocoa powder.

Per serving (1 cup) Calories: 83; Total fat: 2g; Saturated fat: 2g; Carbohydrates: 11g; Sugar: 10g; Fiber: 1g; Protein: 4g

BAKED CINNAMON APPLE CHIPS

Makes 3 Cups • **Prep time:** 20 MINUTES, PLUS 1 HOUR
TO COOL • **Cook time:** 2 HOURS 40 MINUTES

Constipation Aid | Energy Booster | GDM-Friendly | Nausea Relief
Postpartum Recovery | Swelling Relief

Homemade apple chips are easy to make and can satisfy both your sweet and crunchy cravings in a healthy way. Keeping the peel on these fruits retains more fiber content, which can help relieve constipation.

3 large Honeycrisp
apples, cored

¾ teaspoon ground
cinnamon

Pinch ground ginger

1. Preheat the oven to 200°F. Line 2 baking sheets with parchment paper.

2. Using a mandoline or sharp knife, cut the apples horizontally into ⅛-inch-thick rounds.

3. On the prepared baking sheets, arrange the apple rounds in a single layer. Sprinkle with cinnamon and ginger.

4. Bake the apple rounds for 1 hour, then rearrange the position of the baking sheets. Bake for another 1 to 1½ hours, or until the apples appear slightly golden.

5. Turn off the oven and let the apple chips cool inside the oven for 1 hour.

6. Store the completely cooled chips in an airtight container at room temperature for up to 1 week.

SUBSTITUTION TIP: If you don't have apples on hand, swap out the apples for pears. If you don't care for Honeycrisp apples, experiment with other varieties—they will all work well.

Per serving (1 cup): Calories: 118; Total fat: <1g; Saturated fat: <1g; Carbohydrates: 32g; Sugar: 23g; Fiber: 6g; Protein: 1g

ROASTED LENTILS

Serves 6 • Prep time: 5 MINUTES • Cook time: 30 MINUTES

Constipation Aid | Energy Booster | GDM-Friendly | Lactation Support
Nausea Relief | Postpartum Recovery | Swelling Relief

If you are craving a crunchy snack, skip the potato chips and try these roasted lentils instead. Packed with fiber, antioxidants, and plant-based protein, these little legumes will satisfy your craving and help keep you fueled up throughout your day. These lentils also work as a healthy topping on salads or soups.

Cooking spray

1½ cups firm-cooked lentils

½ tablespoon extra-virgin olive oil

Salt

Freshly ground black pepper

1. Preheat the oven to 300°F. Coat a baking sheet with cooking spray.

2. Dry the lentils by patting them with a paper towel.

3. In a medium bowl, combine the lentils, oil, salt, and pepper and toss together.

4. Spread the lentil mixture in an even layer on the prepared baking sheet.

5. Bake for 30 minutes, stirring every 10 minutes, or until lentils are evenly browned.

6. Let cool completely before serving.

SUBSTITUTION TIP: Use garlic powder, turmeric, or cinnamon sugar instead of the salt and pepper.

Per serving (¼ cup): Calories: 67; Total fat: 1g; Saturated fat: <1g; Carbohydrates: 10g; Sugar: <1g; Fiber: 3g; Protein: 5g

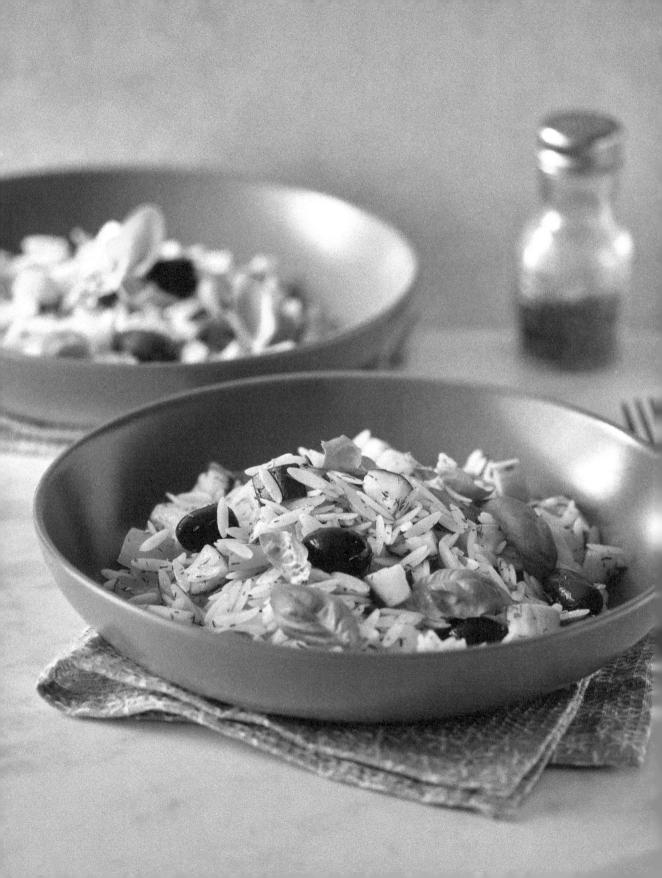

FOUR

SALADS AND SIDES

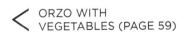

ORZO WITH
VEGETABLES (PAGE 59)

GRILLED CHICKEN, AVOCADO, AND MANGO SALAD

Serves 4 • Prep time: 10 MINUTES
Constipation Aid | GDM-Friendly | Lactation Support
Postpartum Recovery | Quick | Swelling Relief

This refreshing salad is chock-full of important nutrients to nourish your baby. Chicken breast is a simple way to boost protein since most people tolerate it well during pregnancy. If you want a heartier meal, enjoy this salad with a small whole-grain roll.

2 ripe avocados, sliced

2 mangos, diced

½ red onion, thinly sliced

1 head butter lettuce, torn into pieces

⅛ cup macadamia nuts

4 tablespoons extra-virgin olive oil

2 tablespoons apple cider vinegar

Salt

Freshly ground black pepper

12 ounces grilled chicken breast, cut into 1-inch strips

1. In a large bowl, combine the avocados, mangos, red onion, lettuce, and nuts.

2. In a small bowl, whisk together the oil, vinegar, salt, and pepper.

3. Drizzle the oil and vinegar mixture on top of the salad. Toss to combine.

4. Divide the salad among 4 serving plates. Top each salad with 3 ounces of chicken.

MAKE IT EASIER: If you don't have grilled chicken breast on hand, use store-bought rotisserie chicken. This salad also works well without chicken, or you can sub in grilled tofu or another grilled meat substitute.

Per serving (about 1 cup): Calories: 503; Total fat: 31g; Saturated fat: 5g; Carbohydrates: 34g; Sugar: 24g; Fiber: 8g; Protein: 29g

SALMON SALAD WITH DATES

Serves 6 • Prep time: 40 MINUTES • Cook time: 10 MINUTES

Energy Booster | GDM-Friendly | Lactation Support

Postpartum Recovery | Swelling Relief

The combination of salmon, walnuts, dates, and cucumbers makes this salad a superstar pregnancy dish. Eating low-mercury seafood two times a week is recommended during pregnancy and lactation, and salmon is a perfect choice to help check off that box. Loaded with healthy fats, fiber, and antioxidants, this salad will keep you full and energized throughout the day.

Cooking spray

1 (2½-pound) salmon fillet, cut into 6 equal pieces

2 tablespoons extra-virgin olive oil

1 teaspoon salt

½ teaspoon freshly ground black pepper

2 cucumbers, diced

½ cup chopped walnuts

6 pitted Medjool dates, slivered

2 tablespoons minced fresh chives

2 tablespoons freshly squeezed lemon juice

2 cups butter lettuce, torn into pieces

1. Preheat the oven to 350°F. Coat a baking sheet with cooking spray.

2. Place the salmon pieces on the baking sheet and drizzle the oil evenly over the top of each. Season with the salt and pepper.

3. Bake the salmon for 20 minutes, or until cooked through.

4. Meanwhile, in a large bowl, combine the cucumbers, walnuts, dates, chives, and lemon juice and toss to combine.

5. Divide the butter lettuce evenly among 6 serving bowls. Top with the cucumber mixture. Place the baked salmon on top of the cucumbers. Season with salt and pepper, if desired.

MAKE IT EASIER: Use a chilled pre-cooked fillet instead of baking one. This is a great use of leftover salmon.

Per serving (1 cup salad and 1 salmon fillet): Calories: 452; Total fat: 21g; Saturated fat: 3g; Carbohydrates: 23g; Sugar: 18g; Fiber: 3g; Protein: 43g

EDAMAME WITH LEMON VINAIGRETTE

Serves 4 • Prep time: 5 MINUTES

Constipation Aid | GDM-Friendly | Energy Booster | Lactation Support
Nausea Relief | Quick | Swelling Relief

Packed with both flavor and nutrition, edamame (cooked whole soy beans) are a light and nutritious side with plenty of fiber and plant-based protein. They contain a slew of nutrients, like vitamin B_6 and magnesium, that are important for a healthy pregnancy. The addition of lemon may make this dish easier to tolerate if you are dealing with nausea. Make sure to wash your lemon very well before you zest it to help reduce your risk of experiencing food-borne illness from any bacteria found on the peel.

½ teaspoon grated lemon zest

Juice of ½ lemon

2 tablespoons fresh basil, chopped

2 tablespoons extra-virgin olive oil

2 tablespoons rice vinegar

Pinch salt

Pinch freshly ground black pepper

2 cups frozen unsalted shelled edamame, thawed

½ red bell pepper, finely diced

1. In a medium bowl, combine the lemon zest, lemon juice, basil, oil, vinegar, salt, and black pepper and whisk to combine.

2. Add the edamame and bell pepper to the dressing and stir to combine.

Per serving (½ cup): Calories: 160; Total fat: 10g; Saturated fat: 1g; Carbohydrates: 9g; Sugar: 3g; Fiber: 3g; Protein: 8g

KALE WITH CHICKPEA COUSCOUS

Serves 4 to 6 • Prep time: 5 MINUTES • Cook time: 15 MINUTES
Energy Booster | Lactation Support | One-Pot | Postpartum Recovery | Quick

There is nothing wrong with eating plain old couscous, but you can get so much more nutrition once you add ingredients like greens, chickpeas, and raisins into the mix. This colorful and nutrient-dense dish makes a great side but is balanced enough to be enjoyed as a main dish, too.

1½ cups couscous

6 cups Swiss chard, chopped

3 tablespoons extra-virgin olive oil

1½ tablespoons minced garlic

1⅔ cups canned chickpeas, drained and rinsed

½ cup golden raisins

1. In a large pot, cook the couscous according to the package instructions.

2. Once the couscous is cooked thoroughly, reduce the heat to low.

3. Add the Swiss chard, oil, garlic, chickpeas, and golden raisins to the pot. Stir to combine.

SUBSTITUTION TIP: For an extra boost of nutrition, top this dish with slivered almonds. You can also swap out the couscous for quinoa if you prefer. If you can't find Swiss chard, any leafy green vegetable will do.

Per serving (1 cup): Calories: 504; Total fat: 13g; Saturated fat: 2g; Carbohydrates: 85g; Sugar: 17g; Fiber: 10g; Protein: 15g

MAPLE ROASTED CARROTS

Serves 4 • Prep time: 5 MINUTES • Cook time: 1 HOUR, PLUS 10 MINUTES TO COOL

Lactation Support | Nausea Relief | Postpartum Recovery

Carrots are a natural source of key nutrients, including beta carotene, a carotenoid that is converted to vitamin A in your body. This nutrient helps support the immune system and vision health, and many other aspects of health for you and your baby. But when eating raw carrots just won't cut it, the butter and natural sweetness of this dish will help you get your vegetables.

Cooking spray

2 pounds medium carrots, peeled and cut into 2-inch coins

3 tablespoons unsalted butter, cut into pieces

3 tablespoons extra-virgin olive oil

¼ cup pure maple syrup

1 teaspoon red pepper flakes (optional)

Salt

Freshly ground black pepper

2 tablespoons chopped fresh parsley

1. Preheat the oven to 400°F. Line a baking sheet with foil and coat with cooking spray.

2. Put the carrots on the prepared baking sheet. Top with the butter, oil, maple syrup, red pepper flakes (if using), and a pinch each of salt and black pepper. Toss to coat. Spread out the carrots in an even layer.

3. Bake the carrots for 50 minutes to 1 hour, tossing every 20 minutes, until tender and browned around the edges.

4. Remove the carrots from the oven and let them cool for 10 minutes. Sprinkle the parsley over the carrots before serving.

VARIATION TIP: For a little extra zing, add 2 tablespoons of 100 percent pure orange juice in step 2.

Per serving (½ cup): Calories: 221; Total fat: 9g; Saturated fat: 5g; Carbohydrates: 35g; Sugar: 23g; Fiber: 6g; Protein: 2g

ORZO WITH VEGETABLES

Serves 6 to 8 • Prep time: 10 MINUTES • Cook time: 20 MINUTES

Energy Booster | Lactation Support | Nausea Relief | Postpartum Recovery | Quick

This easy pasta dish is equally delicious hot or cold. Combining veggies with orzo helps get key nutrients into your diet, especially on days when you don't feel up for much.

1 (16-ounce) package orzo pasta

3 tablespoons extra-virgin olive oil

2 yellow squash, diced

2 zucchini, diced

1 red bell pepper, diced

1½ teaspoons dried oregano

2 teaspoons dried dill

¼ cup kalamata olives, sliced

Pinch salt

Pinch freshly ground black pepper

1. In a large pot, cook the orzo according to package instructions. Reserve ¼ cup of the cooking water.

2. Meanwhile, in a medium skillet over medium heat, combine the oil, squash, zucchini, and red bell pepper. Sauté the vegetables for 6 minutes, or until soft.

3. In a large bowl, combine the cooked orzo, sautéed vegetables, oregano, dill, and olives. If the pasta is sticking together, add a little bit of the cooking water.

4. Season with salt and black pepper.

VARIATION TIP: For more protein, add pasteurized feta to the salad in step 3. Let the orzo cool completely before adding the feta to prevent it from melting.

Per serving (about 1 cup): Calories: 379; Total fat: 9g; Saturated fat: 1g; Carbohydrates: 63g; Sugar: 7g; Fiber: 5g; Protein: 11g

CAULIFLOWER AND POTATO MASH

Serves 6 • Prep time: 10 MINUTES • Cook time: 20 MINUTES

Energy Booster | Freezer-Friendly | Nausea Relief | One-Pot | Postpartum Recovery

Mashed potatoes are a wonderful comfort food—especially if you are feeling nausea or fatigue. Adding cauliflower to this dish boosts nutrition by providing choline, vitamin C, and other key nutrients. Keeping the skin on the potatoes gives this dish a fiber boost that can help relieve constipation naturally.

2 pounds white or yellow potatoes, cut into 2-inch pieces

4 cups cauliflower florets

2 cups vegetable broth

Salt

2 tablespoons unsalted butter

1 cup 2 percent milk, plus more as needed

1 tablespoon chopped fresh parsley

Freshly ground black pepper

1. In a large pot, combine the potatoes, cauliflower, broth, and salt and bring to a boil. Once it is boiling, reduce the heat to low, cover, and simmer the potatoes for 25 minutes, or until a knife passes through them with no resistance.

2. Drain the potatoes and cauliflower, then return them to the pot.

3. Add the butter and milk to the potatoes and cauliflower. Mash until the mixture reaches your desired consistency.

4. Top with parsley and pepper before serving.

SUBSTITUTION TIP: Try adding other vegetables to sneak in more nutrients. Carrots can give mashed potatoes a slightly sweet flavor and boost the nutritional value of the dish.

MAKE IT EASIER: If you want to keep a batch of this on hand for busy nights, let the dish cool completely, then store in an airtight container in the freezer for up to 3 months.

Per serving (½ cup): Calories: 176; Total fat: 5g; Saturated fat: 3g; Carbohydrates: 29g; Sugar: 6g; Fiber: 5g; Protein: 6g

SWEET AND SOUR BROCCOLI SALAD WITH CASHEWS

Serves 4 • **Prep time:** 5 MINUTES • **Cook time:** 2 MINUTES

Constipation Aid | Postpartum Recovery | Quick

Even if you don't love broccoli, the flavorful dressing in this salad may help you look at it in a new light. With the addition of ingredients like cashews, you can feel confident that you are getting plenty of the healthy fats and protein you and your baby need—especially if this salad is the only thing that tastes good to you at this stage.

1½ cups broccoli florets

1 tablespoon water

½ tablespoon soy sauce

2 teaspoons pure maple syrup

1½ teaspoons rice vinegar

1 cup snap peas

¼ cup cashews, chopped

1 scallion, green part only, thinly sliced

1. In a medium microwave-safe bowl, combine the broccoli and water. Cover with a microwave-safe plate and microwave on high for 2 minutes, then let the broccoli cool.

2. Meanwhile, in a small bowl, whisk together the soy sauce, maple syrup, and vinegar.

3. In a medium bowl, combine the cooked broccoli, snap peas, cashews, scallion, and the dressing. Toss to coat before serving.

SUBSTITUTION TIP: Try adding sriracha sauce, sesame seeds, or sesame oil in step 2.

Per serving (¾ cup): Calories: 74; Total fat: 4g; Saturated fat: 1g; Carbohydrates: 8g; Sugar: 4g; Fiber: 2g; Protein: 3g

CAPRESE PASTA SALAD

Serves 4 • **Prep time:** 5 MINUTES • **Cook time:** 10 MINUTES,
PLUS 5 MINUTES TO COOL

Energy Booster | Lactation Support | Nausea Relief | One-Pot | Quick

Pasta gets a bad rap, but this pregnancy favorite can be part of a healthy pregnancy diet. Adding veggies and protein-packed cheese makes this dish nutritionally balanced and gives you necessary energy. When preparing this dish, make sure the noodles aren't hot, as they will cause the cheese to melt and clump. Keep leftovers covered in the refrigerator for up to 3 days and enjoy warm or cold.

1 (16-ounce) package fusilli or rotini pasta

2 large tomatoes, diced

½ red onion, thinly sliced (optional)

4 tablespoons chopped fresh basil

2 teaspoons balsamic vinegar

3 tablespoons extra-virgin olive oil

½ cup cubed (½-inch) pasteurized mozzarella cheese

Salt

Freshly ground black pepper

1. In a large pot, cook the pasta according to package instructions. Drain and let cool completely, about 5 minutes.

2. In a large bowl, combine the cooked pasta, tomatoes, red onion (if using), basil, vinegar, oil, and cheese. Season with salt and pepper, then toss until the ingredients are well combined.

Per serving (1 cup): Calories: 378; Total fat: 15g; Saturated fat: 4g; Carbohydrates: 48g; Sugar: 5g; Fiber: 3g; Protein: 12g

AVOCADO, ALMOND, AND PEAR SALAD

Serves 4 • **Prep time:** 5 MINUTES

Constipation Aid | GDM-Friendly | Lactation Support
Postpartum Recovery | Quick | Swelling Relief

If you are looking for relief from constipation, this salad is for you, as pear and avocado will help support a healthy gut. Pair them with a simple lemony dressing and crunchy almonds and you've got a tasty way to stay regular.

2 pears, unpeeled, cut into 1-inch cubes

2 ripe avocados, cut into 1-inch cubes

Juice of 1 lemon, divided

2 tablespoons extra-virgin olive oil, divided

Pinch salt

Pinch freshly ground black pepper

4 ounces unsalted sliced almonds, divided

1. Divide the pears and avocados evenly among 4 plates.

2. Top each salad evenly with the lemon juice and oil. Season with salt and pepper.

3. Sprinkle the almonds evenly on top of each salad before serving.

SUBSTITUTION TIP: Feel free to swap out the almonds for crushed macadamia nuts, if desired.

Per serving (1 cup): Calories: 397; Total fat: 32g; Saturated fat: 3g; Carbohydrates: 25g; Sugar: 10g; Fiber: 11g; Protein: 8g

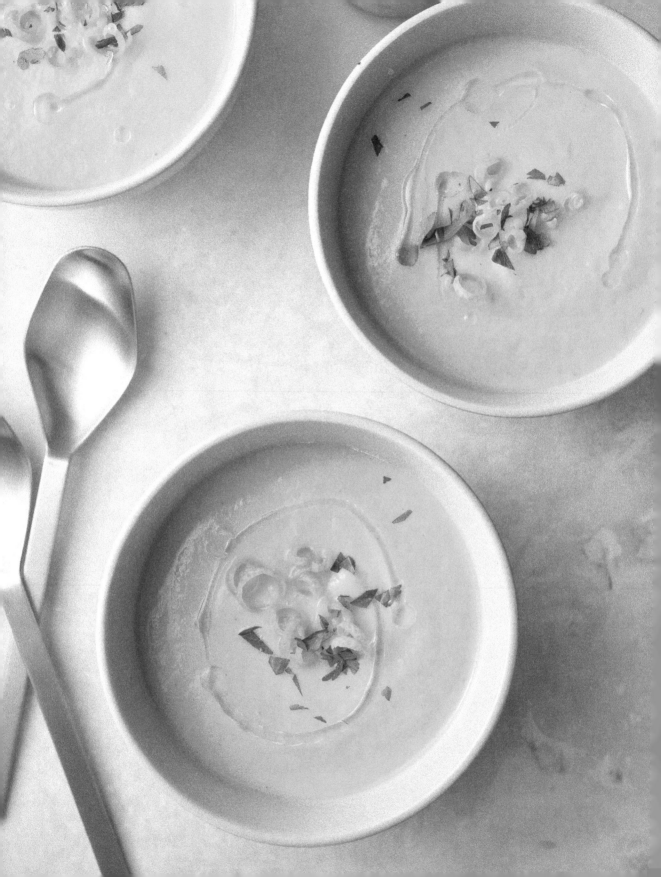

FIVE

SOUPS AND STEWS

< CHILLED GINGER
CARROT SOUP (PAGE 68)

CREAMY CAULIFLOWER SOUP

Serves 4 • Prep time: 10 MINUTES • Cook time: 50 MINUTES,
PLUS 10 MINUTES TO COOL

Freezer-Friendly | GDM-Friendly | Lactation Support
Nausea Relief | Postpartum Recovery

Creamy soups are often comforting when you are not feeling your best. And this soup not only helps keep you hydrated, but it also is a source of protein, calcium, choline, and a slew of other pregnancy-fueling nutrients that are sometimes hard to get, thanks to those pesky side effects.

Cooking spray

1 large head cauliflower (about 2 pounds), cut into florets

3 tablespoons extra-virgin olive oil, divided

Salt

1 medium yellow onion, chopped

2 tablespoons minced garlic

2 cups vegetable broth

2 cups 2 percent milk

1 tablespoon freshly squeezed lemon juice

1 teaspoon ground nutmeg

Freshly ground black pepper

1. Preheat the oven to 425°F. Spray a baking sheet with cooking spray.

2. Put the cauliflower on the prepared baking sheet and toss with 2 tablespoons of oil and a pinch of salt. Then arrange the cauliflower in a single layer.

3. Bake the cauliflower for 15 minutes. Then remove the baking sheet from the oven and stir the cauliflower. Bake for an additional 15 minutes.

4. Meanwhile, in a large pot, heat the remaining 1 tablespoon of oil over medium heat. Add the onion and cook, stirring occasionally, until the onion has softened, about 5 minutes.

5. Add the garlic and cook, stirring constantly, for 1 minute, or until fragrant. Add the broth and milk and stir until combined.

6. Transfer the baked cauliflower to the pot, bring soup to a boil, and then reduce the heat to low and simmer for 20 minutes. Turn off the heat.

7. Add the lemon juice, nutmeg, and pepper.

8. Allow soup to cool for 10 minutes, then transfer it to a blender. Blend until smooth.

MAKE IT EASIER: You may have to blend this soup in batches depending on how much liquid your blender can hold. Freeze one or more batches of this soup by storing it in an airtight container for up to 6 months.

Per serving (1 cup): Calories: 235; Total fat: 14g; Saturated fat: 3g; Carbohydrates: 22g; Sugar: 12g; Fiber: 5g; Protein: 9g

CHILLED GINGER CARROT SOUP

Serves 4 to 6 • **Prep time:** 10 MINUTES • **Cook time:** 30 MINUTES,
PLUS 2 HOURS TO CHILL

GDM-Friendly | Lactation Support | Nausea Relief | Swelling Relief

Chilled soup can sometimes be just what the doctor ordered if you are having trouble keeping food down. And it can also be a lifesaver on busy days when you need some nutrition but don't have time to sit down for a meal. The addition of ginger in this soup can help alleviate nausea symptoms, and it may also help support breast milk supply.

2 tablespoons
extra-virgin olive oil

1 yellow onion, diced

1½ pounds carrots,
peeled and sliced

Pinch salt

1 tablespoon fresh
ginger, minced

¼ teaspoon orange zest

3 cups vegetable broth

1 cup 2 percent milk

1 teaspoon dried thyme

1. In a large pot over medium-high heat, heat the oil until sizzling.

2. Reduce the heat to medium, add the onion, and sauté them for about 3 minutes. Add the carrots and salt and cook for another 5 minutes, or until the carrots begin to soften.

3. Add the ginger, orange zest, and broth. Bring the soup to a boil, then reduce the heat to low. Stir in the milk and thyme, cover, and simmer for 20 minutes.

4. Remove the soup from the heat. Working in batches, blend the soup in a blender until smooth.

5. Refrigerate for about 2 hours before serving.

SUBSTITUTION TIP: To serve the soup hot, skip step 5. If you want a dairy-free soup, swap out the milk for an additional cup of vegetable broth.

Per serving (1 cup): Calories: 187; Total fat: 9g; Saturated fat: 2g; Carbohydrates: 25g; Sugar: 14g; Fiber: 5g; Protein: 4g

CHEESY TORTELLINI SOUP

Serves 4 • Prep time: 5 MINUTES • Cook time: 10 MINUTES

Energy Booster | Lactation Support | One-Pot | Postpartum Recovery | Quick

This soup is surprisingly easy to make, yet it is utterly satisfying and packed with important nutrients for a healthy pregnancy. Using premade tortellini is an effortless way to boost protein, and tomatoes and spinach offer vitamins and minerals, like folate and vitamin C.

4 cups low-sodium vegetable broth

10 ounces fresh cheese tortellini

1 (14.5-ounce) can diced tomatoes

1 teaspoon dried Italian seasoning blend

3 cups spinach, chopped

2 tablespoons grated Parmesan cheese

Pinch salt

Pinch freshly ground black pepper

1. In a medium pot over medium-high heat, bring the broth to a boil.

2. Add the tortellini and cook until almost tender, 3 to 5 minutes.

3. Add the tomatoes with their juices and Italian seasoning and cook for 2 minutes.

4. Add the spinach and cook for 4 minutes, or until it has wilted.

5. Divide the soup among 4 bowls. Sprinkle Parmesan cheese over each serving and season with salt and pepper.

SUBSTITUTION TIP: If you prefer plain pasta, swap out the tortellini for farfalle (or bowties), and cook them in the broth for 9 minutes or until cooked to your liking. For more nutrition, you can also add other vegetables, like frozen diced carrots and peas.

Per serving (1 cup): Calories: 274; Total fat: 6g; Saturated fat: 3g; Carbohydrates: 42g; Sugar: 5g; Fiber: 4g; Protein: 13g

LENTIL CARROT SOUP

Serves 4 to 6 • Prep time: 20 MINUTES • Cook time: 1 HOUR 15 MINUTES

Constipation Aid | Energy Booster | Freezer-Friendly

Lactation Support | Postpartum Recovery

Easy, inexpensive, and delicious, this vegan-friendly soup is loaded with good-for-you nutrients like folate, beta carotene, and fiber. Plus, this soup freezes well, so you can double up on your batch and freeze the leftovers.

2 tablespoons extra-virgin olive oil

1 cup yellow onion, chopped

1 cup chopped carrots

2 tablespoons minced garlic

2 tablespoons tomato paste

5 cups reduced-sodium vegetable broth

1 cup dry lentils, rinsed and picked over

1 teaspoon dried dill

Salt

Freshly ground black pepper

1. In a large pot, heat the oil over medium-high heat. Add the onion and carrots and cook for 4 minutes, or until the onions are translucent.

2. Add the garlic and tomato paste and cook for 2 minutes, or until the garlic is fragrant.

3. Add the broth, lentils, and dill. Bring the soup to a boil. Reduce the heat to low, cover, and simmer for 40 minutes.

4. Season with salt and pepper before serving.

VARIATION TIP: If you can tolerate spice, add some heat to this soup by adding a sprinkle of cayenne pepper before serving.

MAKE IT EASIER: You can freeze one or more batches of this soup by storing it in an airtight container for up to 6 months.

Per serving (1 cup): Calories: 290; Total fat: 8g; Saturated fat: 1g; Carbohydrates: 43g; Sugar: 7g; Fiber: 7g; Protein: 14g

WHITE BEAN CHICKEN CHILI

Serves 4 to 6 • **Prep time:** 5 MINUTES • **Cook time:** 15 MINUTES

Constipation Aid | Energy Booster | Freezer-Friendly | GDM-Friendly

Lactation Support | One-Pot | Postpartum Recovery

This satisfying chili uses dark meat chicken for extra iron, a nutrient that most pregnant people need more of, especially during the second trimester. It's also packed with other important nutrients, like vitamin B_{12}, choline, and high-quality protein. Best of all, it is quick and simple to make on busy weeknights.

5 cups chicken broth

3½ cups cooked and shredded dark meat chicken

2 (15-ounce) cans Great Northern beans

2 cups store-bought salsa verde

2 teaspoons ground cumin

1 jalapeño, diced (optional)

1 ripe avocado, thinly sliced

1 cup cherry tomatoes, quartered

1 tablespoon shredded cheddar cheese (optional)

Freshly ground black pepper

1. In a large pot, combine the broth, chicken, beans with their liquid, salsa verde, cumin, and jalapeño (if using) and bring to a boil over high heat.

2. Once the soup is boiling, reduce the heat to medium-low and simmer for 10 minutes.

3. Top each serving with avocado, cherry tomatoes, cheese (if using), and black pepper.

SUBSTITUTION TIP: If you want a milder flavor, omit the cumin and add just 1 cup of the salsa verde.

MAKE IT EASIER: You can freeze one or more batches of this soup. Simply complete steps 1 and 2 as directed, then freeze the soup in an airtight container for up to 6 months. After thawing and reheating, top with avocado, tomatoes, cheese, and black pepper just before serving.

Per serving (1 cup): Calories: 559; Total fat: 18g; Saturated fat: 4g; Carbohydrates: 53g; Sugar: 7g; Fiber: 15g; Protein: 48g

CHICKEN SAUSAGE, CHICKPEA, AND KALE SOUP

Serves 4 to 6 • Prep time: 15 MINUTES • Cook time: 20 MINUTES

Constipation Aid | Freezer-Friendly | GDM-Friendly | One-Pot
Postpartum Recovery | Quick | Swelling Relief

This hearty soup is a stick-to-your-ribs option that goes well with a piece of crusty bread on a cozy night in. Full of folic acid, fiber, vitamin B_6, and a slew of other nutrients, this soup is sure to please and nourish both you and your growing baby.

1 tablespoon extra-virgin olive oil

1 medium onion, chopped

1 (19-ounce) package natural chicken sausage (made without nitrates), cut into 1-inch pieces

1 tablespoon minced garlic

1 (16-ounce) can crushed tomatoes

1 (16-ounce) can chickpeas, drained and rinsed

4 cups low-sodium chicken broth

1 bunch kale, chopped

Salt

1 teaspoon freshly ground black pepper

1. In a large pot, heat the oil over medium heat. Add the onion and cook for 5 minutes, or until translucent.

2. Add the sausage and cook for 5 minutes, or until it begins to brown.

3. Reduce the heat to medium-low and add the garlic. Cook for 2 minutes, or until fragrant.

4. Add the tomatoes with their juices, chickpeas, and broth, and bring to a boil. Then reduce the heat to medium-low and simmer for 15 minutes.

5. Add the kale and simmer for 5 minutes more. Season with salt and pepper before serving.

SUBSTITUTION TIP: Use pork, turkey, or vegan sausage if you prefer.

MAKE IT EASIER: You can make multiple batches of this soup and freeze it in an airtight container for up to 4 months.

Per serving (1 cup): Calories: 422; Total fat: 19g; Saturated fat: 5g; Carbohydrates: 30g; Sugar: 9g; Fiber: 8g; Protein: 35g

EGG DROP SOUP

Serves 4 to 6 • Prep time: 5 MINUTES • Cook time: 10 MINUTES

GDM-Friendly | Lactation Support | One-Pot | Postpartum Recovery | Quick

Eggs are one of the best sources of choline, a key nutrient for a baby's brain development. Egg drop soup is a delicious way to take in this nutrient, but when ordering it at a restaurant, it can be loaded with sodium. Making your own is incredibly easy and just as delicious! The addition of spinach makes this version even more nutritious.

3 eggs

4 cups low-sodium vegetable broth

2 tablespoons cornstarch

1 teaspoon ground ginger

¼ teaspoon garlic powder

1 cup spinach, chopped

3 scallions, both white and green parts, thinly sliced

Salt

Freshly ground black pepper

1 teaspoon soy sauce (optional)

1. In a small bowl, whisk the eggs until combined. Set aside.

2. In a medium saucepan, whisk together the broth, cornstarch, ginger, and garlic powder. Then bring the mixture to a boil over high heat.

3. Once it reaches a boil, reduce the heat to medium-low and simmer for 5 minutes, stirring occasionally.

4. Slowly pour the eggs into the soup, whisking continuously.

5. Add the spinach and simmer for 5 minutes, or until the spinach has wilted. Remove the pan from the heat.

6. Stir in the scallions, then add salt, pepper, and soy sauce (if using).

SUBSTITUTION TIP: Replace the spinach with bok choy, if desired. Or, to add fiber and flavor, add ½ cup of mushrooms or corn kernels in step 5 to enrich the flavor and fiber content.

Per serving (1 cup): Calories: 82; Total fat: 4g; Saturated fat: 1g; Carbohydrates: 7g; Sugar: 2g; Fiber: <1g; Protein: 5g

CLASSIC CHICKEN NOODLE SOUP

Serves 6 to 8 • **Prep time:** 15 MINUTES • **Cook time:** 40 MINUTES

Nausea Relief | One-Pot | Postpartum Recovery

What's better than a bowl of chicken noodle soup when you need a pick-me-up? Chicken noodle soup is the ultimate comfort food. It can help maintain hydration and electrolyte levels when you can't stomach many other food options. Although it is a simple recipe, this dish should not be underestimated in terms of how much it can help you feel energized and nourished.

8 cups chicken broth

4 boneless, skinless chicken thighs

2 dill sprigs

1½ cups ½-inch carrot slices

1 cup ½-inch celery slices

Salt

Freshly ground black pepper

2 cups cooked whole-grain farfalle or bowtie noodles

1. In a large pot over high heat, bring the broth to a boil. Add the chicken and dill and cook for 10 minutes, or until the chicken begins to brown.

2. Add the carrots and celery. Stir and continue cooking for 10 more minutes, or until the chicken is cooked through.

3. Reduce the heat to medium-low and let the soup simmer for at least 15 minutes. Remove the chicken from the soup, place it on a cutting board or plate, and shred it with a fork. Return the shredded chicken to the pot.

4. To serve, place an equal portion of cooked noodles in the bottom of 6 serving bowls. Ladle the soup over the noodles and season with salt and pepper.

SUBSTITUTION TIP: For extra protein, use chickpea-based noodles instead.

Per serving (1 cup): Calories: 192; Total fat: 4g; Saturated fat: 1g; Carbohydrates: 19g; Sugar: 4g; Fiber: 2g; Protein: 20g

MISO AND VEGGIE SOUP

Serves 4 to 6 • Prep time: 5 MINUTES • Cook time: 10 MINUTES
GDM-Friendly | Nausea Relief | One-Pot | Postpartum Recovery | Quick

This miso soup is nourishing and healing by nature, thanks to the amino acids it contains, and has a satisfying umami flavor. Nori sheets add iodine, an important nutrient that supports a baby's brain health. The addition of tofu to this recipe helps support bone strength by providing a boost of calcium. Make sure to not heat the soup too much when you add the miso paste, as most live probiotics become inactive above 100°F.

8 cups vegetable or mushroom broth

2 sheets nori (dried seaweed), cut into large ½-inch-by-1-inch rectangles

1 cup sliced mushrooms

1 bunch scallions, both white and green parts, chopped

½ cup firm tofu, cubed

6 tablespoons miso paste

1 tablespoon hot water

1. In a medium pot over low heat, bring the broth to a simmer.

2. Add the nori, mushrooms, and scallions and cook for 5 minutes. Add the tofu and cook for 2 minutes more. Remove the saucepan from heat and set aside.

3. In a small bowl, combine the miso paste and hot water and mix well.

4. Stir the miso mixture into the soup before serving.

Per serving (1 cup): Calories: 134; Total fat: 5g; Saturated fat: 1g; Carbohydrates: 14g; Sugar: 5g; Fiber: 3g; Protein: 11g

BAKED POTATO SOUP

Serves 4 • Prep time: 15 MINUTES • Cook time: 25 MINUTES
Energy Booster | Freezer-Friendly | Lactation Support
Nausea Relief | Postpartum Recovery

Baked potato soup is a nourishing, filling option for those days when you just feel too busy to eat. If nausea strikes, this soup may be the perfect solution, thanks to its hearty and comforting healthy carbs. Potatoes contain potassium, and the addition of milk gives this soup a boost of protein. Plus, the Greek yogurt gives this soup some probiotics to help support healthy gut flora.

1 tablespoon unsalted butter, softened

⅔ cup all-purpose flour

7 cups 2 percent milk

4 large pre-baked potatoes, peeled and cubed

2 bunches scallions, both white and green parts, chopped

1 cup shredded cheddar cheese

1 cup 2 percent plain Greek yogurt

Salt

Freshly ground black pepper

4 slices pre-cooked turkey bacon, crumbled (optional)

1. In a large soup pot, melt the butter over medium heat. Whisk in the flour until smooth. Gradually stir in the milk, whisking constantly until thickened.

2. Stir in the potatoes and scallions.

3. Bring the soup to a boil, stirring frequently. Then reduce the heat to low and simmer for 12 minutes, or until the soup is heated through.

4. Add the cheese, yogurt, salt, and pepper. Cook for 5 minutes more, stirring occasionally.

5. Divide evenly among 4 serving bowls. Top each serving with turkey bacon (if using).

VARIATION TIP: Try garnishing this soup with chopped fresh chives if you can tolerate them.

MAKE IT EASIER: This is a great meal to make if you have leftover baked potatoes. You can also make one or more batches of this soup and freeze it in airtight containers for up to 4 months.

Per serving (1 cup): Calories: 513; Total fat: 15g; Saturated fat: 9g; Carbohydrates: 71g; Sugar: 19g; Fiber: 6g; Protein: 25g

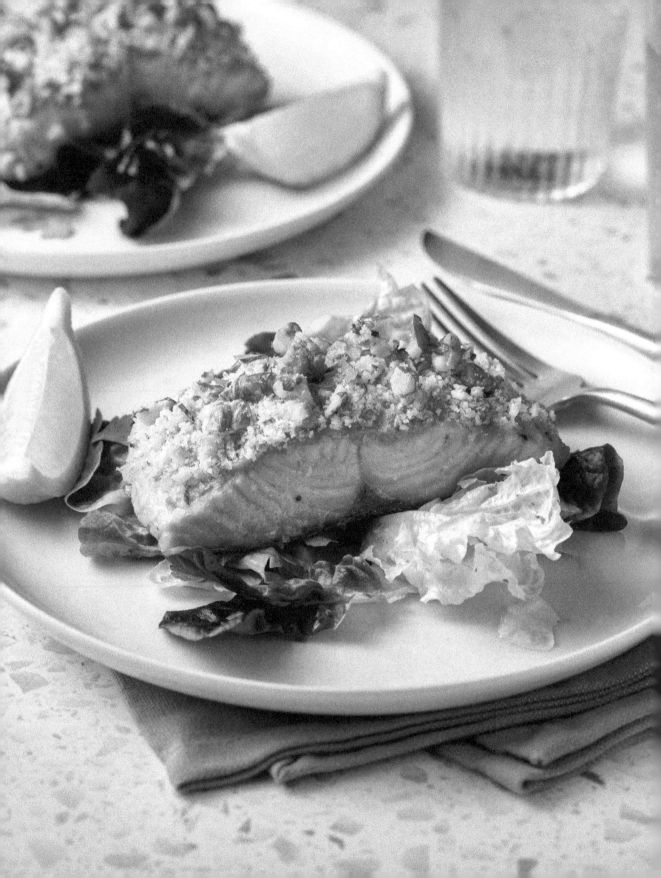

ENTRÉES

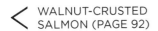

WALNUT-CRUSTED
SALMON (PAGE 92)

GINGER TOFU CITRUS BOWL

Serves 4 • **Prep time:** 5 MINUTES • **Cook time:** 10 MINUTES

GDM-Friendly | Lactation Support | Nausea Relief | Postpartum Recovery | Quick

For days when you feel queasy and you are having a hard time figuring out what to make for dinner, this dish is quick, easy, and loaded with ginger to help give you some relief. Tofu is typically easy to tolerate and gives your body key nutrients like protein and calcium.

10 ounces extra-firm tofu

2½ tablespoons marmalade

2½ tablespoons soy sauce

5 tablespoons water

1½ tablespoons extra-virgin olive oil

1½ tablespoons minced garlic

2½ teaspoons minced fresh ginger

2 cups chopped bok choy

2½ tablespoons unsalted raw cashews

1. Wrap the tofu in paper towels and place something heavy on top, such as a cast-iron skillet or a textbook. Set aside and allow to drain for about 5 minutes.

2. In a small bowl, whisk together the marmalade, soy sauce, and water. Set aside.

3. In a medium skillet, heat the oil over high heat for about 2 minutes, or until sizzling.

4. Meanwhile, unwrap the tofu and cut into 1-inch cubes. Set aside.

5. Once the oil is sizzling, put the garlic and ginger into the skillet and cook for 2 minutes, or until fragrant.

6. Add the tofu cubes and stir-fry gently for 3 minutes.

7. Add the bok choy and cook for 2 minutes more, or until it begins to brown.

8. Stir in the marmalade sauce and cook for 2 minutes.

9. Divide evenly among 4 serving bowls and top with cashews before serving.

SUBSTITUTION TIP: Serve over brown rice to increase your intake of whole grains. If you can tolerate it, consider adding a sprinkle of red pepper flakes to the marmalade sauce. If you can't find bok choy, use spinach.

Per serving (½ cup): Calories: 206; Total fat: 11g; Saturated fat: 2g; Carbohydrates: 16g; Sugar: 7g; Fiber: 2g; Protein: 10g

MEXICAN-INSPIRED BAKED POTATOES

Serves 4 • **Prep time:** 10 MINUTES • **Cook time:** 1 HOUR

Constipation Aid | Energy Booster | Lactation Support | Postpartum Recovery

Potatoes are a natural source of healthy carbohydrates, potassium, and fiber, especially if you eat the skin. Using a baked potato as a vessel for yummy, sensible toppings lets you enjoy delicious flavors without the empty calories.

4 medium russet potatoes

1 tablespoon extra-virgin olive oil

1 small Spanish onion, diced

1 (15-ounce) can black beans, rinsed and drained

1 (15-ounce) can diced tomatoes

½ cup salsa

1½ cups canned sweet corn

4 tablespoons 2 percent plain Greek yogurt

Salt

Freshly ground black pepper

1. Preheat the oven to 400°F.

2. To prepare the potatoes, scrub them and pat them dry. Using a fork, poke holes in each potato. Place the potatoes on the oven rack and bake for 1 hour.

3. Meanwhile, in a large skillet, heat the oil over medium heat for 2 minutes, or until sizzling. Add the onion and sauté for 5 minutes, or until translucent.

4. Add the black beans, tomatoes with their juices, salsa, and corn. Reduce the heat to medium-low and simmer for 10 minutes.

5. When the potatoes are finished baking, remove them from the oven. Cut them lengthwise, but not all the way through. Squeeze the sides and fluff the inside with a fork, leaving the potato skin intact.

6. Top each potato with the black bean mixture. Dollop with 1 tablespoon of Greek yogurt. Season with salt and pepper.

VARIATION TIP: Add your favorite toppings, like shredded cheese, black olives, or diced avocado.

Per serving (1 loaded potato) Calories: 398; Total fat: 5g; Saturated fat: 1g; Carbohydrates: 76g; Sugar: 10g; Fiber: 15g; Protein: 15g

TEX-MEX NAAN PIZZAS

Serves 3 • Prep time: 5 MINUTES • Cook time: 30 MINUTES

Constipation Aid | GDM-Friendly | Energy Booster | Postpartum Recovery

Are you looking for a good-for-you alternative to cheesy pizza? Look no further. This quick pizza uses mashed avocado as the "sauce" so you can take advantage of the carbohydrates, potassium, and healthy fats in avocados, a genuine superfood. Black beans give this dish a boost of fiber to help keep things moving. Naan, a delicious Indian flatbread, is available in most grocery chains and on Amazon, but if you can't find it, use any flatbread you're able to find.

1 tablespoon extra-virgin olive oil

⅓ white onion, diced

1 green bell pepper, diced

½ teaspoon ground cumin

¼ teaspoon salt

½ teaspoon freshly ground black pepper

1 (15-ounce) can black beans, rinsed and drained

1 cup fresh or frozen corn kernels

6 (6- to 7-inch) naan

1 cup chopped avocado

2 tomatoes, diced (optional)

2 tablespoons fresh cilantro (optional)

1. Preheat the oven to 350°F. Line 2 baking sheets with parchment paper.

2. In a large skillet, heat the oil over medium-high heat for 2 minutes, or until sizzling. Add the onion, bell pepper, cumin, salt, and black pepper and sauté for 10 minutes.

3. Add the black beans and corn and cook for another 4 minutes.

4. Arrange the naan on the prepared baking sheets. Bake for 10 to 15 minutes, or until they are toasted.

5. In a small bowl, use a fork to mash the avocado. Spread the avocado, then the bean mixture on each toasted naan. Top with tomatoes and cilantro (if using).

MAKE IT EASIER: Wait to bake the naan until the onion, bell pepper, and cumin are almost finished cooking. If the naan comes out of the oven too early, it will become chewy.

Per serving (2 small pizzas): Calories: 825; Total fat: 22g; Saturated fat: 4g; Carbohydrates: 133g; Sugar: 9g; Fiber: 19g; Protein: 28g

LEMONY RICOTTA PASTA WITH CRUSHED PISTACHIOS

Serves 4 • Prep time: 5 MINUTES • Cook time: 20 MINUTES

Energy Booster | GDM-Friendly | Lactation Support | Nausea Relief
One-Pot | Postpartum Recovery | Quick

On those nights when you want something satisfying but you don't want to be standing over a hot stove all evening, this is the dish to make. The ricotta cheese is mild and usually easy to tolerate for the nauseated crowd. Even though this dinner is vegetarian, it packs a punch in the protein department.

1 (16-ounce) package penne pasta

1 cup whole milk ricotta cheese, pasteurized

½ cup grated Parmesan cheese

½ cup freshly squeezed lemon juice

1½ teaspoons minced garlic

Pinch salt

Pinch freshly ground black pepper

¼ cup arugula

¼ cup unsalted shelled and crushed pistachios

4 fresh basil leaves (optional)

1. In a large pot, cook the pasta according to package instructions. Reserve 1 cup of the pasta water, then drain and set aside.

2. In the same pot over medium-low heat, combine the ricotta cheese, Parmesan cheese, lemon juice, garlic, ½ cup of reserved pasta water, the salt, and pepper. Cook for about 5 minutes, or until the cheese begins to melt. Add more water if the sauce is too thick.

3. Add the cooked pasta to the sauce and stir to combine. Add the arugula and cook, stirring until the arugula has wilted, about 3 minutes. Remove the pot from the heat.

4. Divide among 4 serving bowls. Top each with pistachios and a basil leaf (if using).

SUBSTITUTION TIP: If you can tolerate it, add a sprinkle of red pepper flakes for a kick. For extra fiber and protein, swap out the pasta for a lentil or chickpea pasta. Just keep in mind that the cook time may be less.

Per serving (about 1 cup): Calories: 622; Total fat: 15g; Saturated fat: 7g; Carbohydrates: 96g; Sugar: 6g; Fiber: 5g; Protein: 25g

VEGAN BUDDHA BOWL

Serves 4 • Prep time: 10 MINUTES • Cook time: 20 MINUTES

Constipation Aid | Energy Booster | GDM-Friendly | Lactation Support

Postpartum Recovery | Quick | Swelling Relief

Loaded with plant-based ingredients that help support your pregnancy, this one-bowl meal is delicious and easy to make. Kale gives this bowl some folate to support your baby's spinal cord development, while the chickpeas add anti-oxidants and fiber to help regulate healthy bowel movements.

1 cup quinoa, rinsed

1 (15-ounce) can chick-peas, drained, rinsed, and patted dry

¼ cup water

1 large bunch dinosaur (lacinato) kale, torn into large pieces

½ cup tahini

1 teaspoon minced garlic

Juice of ¼ lemon

Salt

Freshly ground black pepper

1. Cook the quinoa according to package instructions.

2. Evenly divide the cooked quinoa and chickpeas among 4 serving bowls.

3. In a medium saucepan over high heat, bring the water to a boil. Then reduce the heat to medium-low.

4. Using a steamer basket, steam the kale for 2 minutes. Remove the pan from the heat. Place the steamed kale on top of the quinoa in each bowl.

5. In a small bowl, whisk together the tahini, garlic, water, lemon juice, salt, and pepper. Drizzle the tahini mixture over the top of each serving.

SUBSTITUTION TIP: This recipe calls for dinosaur kale, a heartier, darker green that stands up well to cooking. However, you can use regular green or red kale if you prefer. If you're short on time or energy, buy pre-cooked quinoa in the frozen food section. Feel free to swap out the quinoa for rice if that's what you have available.

Per serving (1 cup): Calories: 605; Total fat: 27g; Saturated fat: 3g; Carbohydrates: 72g; Sugar: 9g; Fiber: 17g; Protein: 22g

CHICKEN AND QUINOA CASSEROLE WITH BROCCOLI

Serves 4 • **Prep time:** 10 MINUTES • **Cook time:** 55 MINUTES

Energy Booster | Freezer-Friendly | Lactation Support
Nausea Relief | Postpartum Recovery

If you are looking for easy dishes to make before your baby comes, this recipe is for you. Using quinoa instead of rice gives this dish an extra boost of protein, B vitamins, fiber, and antioxidants, and the broccoli adds pregnancy-fueling iron and folate.

Cooking spray

1 cup uncooked quinoa

1 tablespoon extra-virgin olive oil

1 pound boneless, skinless chicken breasts, diced into 1-inch cubes

1 tablespoon minced garlic

1 (14.5-ounce) can low-sodium chicken broth

Salt

Freshly ground black pepper

¼ teaspoon dried thyme

2½ cups frozen broccoli florets, thawed

1 cup shredded cheddar cheese

1. Preheat the oven to 400°F. Coat the inside of a 9-by-13-inch baking dish with cooking spray.

2. Rinse the quinoa with cold water until the water runs clear.

3. In a large skillet, heat the oil over medium-high heat for 2 minutes, or until sizzling. Add the chicken and cook, stirring occasionally, for 4 minutes, or until it begins to brown.

4. Add the garlic and sauté for 1 minute, or until fragrant.

5. Add the broth, quinoa, salt, pepper, and thyme to the skillet and stir to combine. Remove from the heat.

6. Pour the chicken and quinoa mixture into the prepared baking dish. Bake uncovered for 40 minutes, or until the chicken is cooked through.

7. Remove the baking dish from the oven, but keep the oven on. Add the broccoli to the baking dish and top with cheese. Return the baking dish to the oven and bake for another 5 minutes, or until the cheese has melted.

MAKE IT EASIER: Cool the casserole completely, then cover it tightly and freeze for up to 4 months. To reheat, thaw completely and bake uncovered for 40 minutes at 400°F.

Per serving (1 cup): Calories: 490; Total fat: 19g; Saturated fat: 7g; Carbohydrates: 38g; Sugar: 5g; Fiber: 7g; Protein: 42g

CHEESY BEEF ENCHILADA CASSEROLE

Serves 4 • Prep time: 15 MINUTES • Cook time: 20 MINUTES

Energy Booster | Freezer-Friendly | Lactation Support | Postpartum Recovery

Enchiladas are always a good idea, but turning them into a casserole makes them even better because there's no need to roll them up. Before your baby is born, make and freeze extra batches of this casserole for quick and easy post-partum meals when you are just too tired to cook.

Cooking spray

1 pound lean ground beef

2 bell peppers, thinly sliced

1 (28-ounce) can crushed tomatoes

2 tablespoons ground cumin

Salt

Freshly ground black pepper

8 (6-inch) corn tortillas

1 (15-ounce) can black beans, rinsed and drained

1 cup shredded Mexican cheese blend

1. Preheat the oven to 350°F. Lightly coat the inside of a 9-by-13-inch baking dish with cooking spray.

2. In a large skillet over medium-high heat, cook the ground beef for about 8 minutes, or until browned. Drain the excess fat, return the meat to the skillet, and cook over medium-low heat for 2 minutes.

3. Stir in the bell peppers and cook for about 5 minutes, or until soft.

4. In a large bowl, combine the tomatoes with their juices, cumin, salt, and black pepper. Then spread ½ cup of the seasoned tomatoes in the bottom of the prepared baking dish.

5. Layer 3 tortillas over the tomatoes. Top with half of the black beans, beef, and peppers. Distribute another ½ cup of tomato mixture over the beef and peppers and sprinkle ½ cup of cheese over the tomatoes.

6. Layer 3 more tortillas over the cheese and top with the remaining half of the black beans, as well as the remaining beef and bell pepper and ¼ cup of cheese. Top with remaining 2 tortillas and ¼ cup of cheese.

7. Bake uncovered for 40 minutes, or until the top is golden brown.

SUBSTITUTION TIP: Just before serving, top the casserole with plain Greek yogurt, salsa, or avocados for added flavor and nutrition.

MAKE IT EASIER: Cool the casserole completely, then cover it tightly and freeze for up to 4 months. To reheat, thaw completely and bake uncovered for 40 minutes at 350°F.

Per serving (1 cup): Calories: 661; Total fat: 25g; Saturated fat: 11g; Carbohydrates: 62g; Sugar: 13g; Fiber: 16g; Protein: 50g

QUICK VEGETARIAN "BEEF" LASAGNA

Serves 8 • Prep time: 15 MINUTES • Cook time: 45 MINUTES

Energy Booster | Freezer-Friendly | Lactation Support

One-Pot | Postpartum Recovery

This lasagna is a great way to get your vegetables without sacrificing flavor. Swapping out beef for chopped mushrooms and using whole-grain noodles boosts fiber, antioxidants, and nutrients like vitamin D and niacin. The cheese adds protein and makes this a stick-to-your-ribs meal. Make sure you buy marinara sauce without high-fructose corn syrup.

Cooking spray

1 tablespoon extra-virgin olive oil

16 ounces button mushrooms, washed and finely chopped

1 (25-ounce) jar marinara sauce

6 uncooked whole-grain lasagna noodles

1 (15-ounce) container part-skim ricotta cheese

1 (8-ounce) package shredded mozzarella cheese

½ cup shredded Parmesan cheese

1 tablespoon dried Italian seasoning blend

1. Preheat the oven to 375°F. Lightly coat the inside of a 12-by-8-inch baking dish with cooking spray.

2. In a medium skillet, heat the oil over medium-high heat for 2 minutes, or until sizzling. Add the mushrooms and cook for about 6 minutes, or until soft. Drain any liquid that may have been released from the mushrooms.

3. Remove the skillet from the heat and stir in the marinara sauce until incorporated.

4. Spread a third of the marinara and mushroom sauce over the bottom of the baking dish. Top with 3 uncooked lasagna noodles. Spread half of the ricotta over the noodles and top with half of the mozzarella cheese and half of the Parmesan cheese.

5. Top with another third of the sauce. Add 3 more lasagna noodles, then spread the remaining half of the ricotta on top of the noodles. Top with the remaining third of the sauce and the remaining mozzarella and Parmesan cheeses. Sprinkle Italian seasoning over the top.

6. Cover the lasagna with foil and bake for 40 minutes. Uncover and bake for another 10 minutes, or until the cheese has melted.

SUBSTITUTION TIP: Swap the mushrooms with ground beef if you prefer, or use a vegan meat substitute.

MAKE IT EASIER: Cool the casserole completely, then cover it tightly and freeze for up to 4 months. To reheat, thaw completely and bake uncovered for 40 minutes at 375°F.

Per serving (1 cup): Calories: 312; Total fat: 16g; Saturated fat: 8g; Carbohydrates: 27g; Sugar: 9g; Fiber: 4g; Protein: 22g

WALNUT-CRUSTED SALMON

Serves 4 • Prep time: 10 MINUTES • Cook time: 15 MINUTES

GDM-Friendly | Lactation Support | Quick | Swelling Relief

Healthy fats are extremely important when it comes to a pregnancy diet, but few foods supply the two essential fatty acids our bodies need: DHA and EPA. Fish is packed with these healthy fats, and salmon is typically lower in mercury than other fish. Adding walnuts to this quick and easy baked salmon gives it extra fiber, antioxidants, and more healthy fats, including omega-3 fatty acids.

¼ cup crushed walnuts

2 tablespoons panko bread crumbs

1 tablespoon grated Parmesan cheese

4 (6-ounce) skin-on salmon fillets

Salt

Freshly ground black pepper

2 tablespoons extra-virgin olive oil

1 tablespoon Dijon mustard

1 lemon, quartered (optional)

1 tablespoon chopped fresh parsley (optional)

1. Preheat the oven to 375°F.

2. In a small bowl, combine the walnuts, panko bread crumbs, and Parmesan cheese and stir until evenly combined. Set aside.

3. Lightly season the salmon fillets with salt and pepper on both sides.

4. In a large oven-safe skillet, heat the oil over medium heat for 2 minutes, or until sizzling. Sear the salmon fillets, flesh-side down, for 3 minutes.

5. Turn off the heat and flip the fillets, skin-side down. Brush the tops of each fillet evenly with Dijon mustard. Top each with the walnut breading, pressing it down into the flesh.

6. Transfer the pan to the oven and cook for about 12 minutes, or until salmon flakes easily with a fork and is cooked through.

7. Serve with lemon wedges and parsley (if using).

MAKE IT EASIER: Serve leftover salmon chilled atop a bed of greens the next day.

Per serving (1 salmon fillet): Calories: 289; Total fat: 15g; Saturated fat: 3g; Carbohydrates: 3g; Sugar: <1g; Fiber: 1g; Protein: 34g

STRIP STEAK WITH CARAMELIZED ONIONS

Serves 4 • **Prep time:** 10 MINUTES • **Cook time:** 30 MINUTES

GDM-Friendly | Postpartum Recovery | Swelling Relief

Once a pregnant person enters the second trimester, their need for iron increases. This recipe features steak, which is one of the best sources of iron. The iron found in beef is often better absorbed than plant-based varieties.

2 tablespoons extra-virgin olive oil, divided

2 white onions, sliced

1½ teaspoons brown sugar

½ cup beef broth

1 tablespoon balsamic vinegar

½ teaspoon salt, divided

¼ teaspoon freshly ground black pepper

1 pound sirloin steak, cut into 4 (1-inch) strips

1. In a large skillet, heat 1 tablespoon of oil over medium heat for 2 minutes, or until sizzling. Add the onions and brown sugar. Cook for 15 minutes, stirring constantly, or until onions have caramelized.

2. Add the broth, vinegar, and ¼ teaspoon of salt. Cook, stirring, for 5 minutes more, or until the broth is heated through. Transfer the caramelized onions to a medium bowl.

3. Sprinkle the remaining ¼ teaspoon of salt and the pepper on the steak.

4. In the same pan, heat the remaining 1 tablespoon of oil over medium-high heat. Add the steaks and cook for 5 minutes on each side. Reduce the heat to medium-low, cover, and cook for another 8 minutes, or until the center is no longer pink and the internal temperature reaches 145°F.

5. Transfer the steak to serving plates and top with onions.

MAKE IT EASIER: To make sure the steak is cooked to an internal temperature of 145°F, invest in a quality instant-read meat thermometer.

Per serving (4-ounce steak topped with caramelized onions): Calories: 273; Total fat: 12g; Saturated fat: 3g; Carbohydrates: 7g; Sugar: 4g; Fiber: 1g; Protein: 35g

CHICKEN PICCATA
WITH ZOODLES

Serves 4 • Prep time: 10 MINUTES • Cook time: 25 MINUTES

Constipation Aid | GDM-Friendly | Nausea Relief

Chicken contains key nutrients like protein, choline, and vitamin B_{12}. The fresh lemon juice in this piccata adds a refreshing zing that can help during bouts of nausea and also provides a boost of vitamin C. This version uses zucchini noodles, or "zoodles," to sneak in some extra fiber.

2 boneless, skinless chicken breasts, halved lengthwise

Salt

Freshly ground black pepper

3 tablespoons extra-virgin olive oil

½ cup all-purpose flour

1 cup chicken broth

3 tablespoons freshly squeezed lemon juice

4 tablespoons capers, drained

4 cups frozen zucchini noodles

1 tablespoon chopped fresh parsley (optional)

1. Season both sides of the chicken breasts with salt and pepper.

2. In a large skillet, heat the oil over medium-high heat for 2 minutes, or until sizzling.

3. Meanwhile, put the flour in a medium shallow bowl. Dredge both sides of the chicken with the flour.

4. Once the oil is sizzling, place the chicken in the skillet and cook for 5 minutes on each side, or until browned. Remove the chicken from the skillet and set aside.

5. In the same skillet, combine the broth, lemon juice, and capers. Using a wooden spoon, deglaze the pan by lightly scraping the browned bits from the bottom of the skillet. Reduce the heat to medium-low and simmer for 5 minutes, or until the liquid has reduced slightly.

6. Return the chicken to the skillet and cook for an additional 5 minutes, or until cooked through.

7. Heat the zucchini noodles according to package instructions. Divide the cooked zucchini noodles evenly among 4 serving plates. Place one chicken breast on top of each plate of noodles and spoon the lemon sauce over the chicken. Garnish with parsley (if using).

SUBSTITUTION TIP: Serve with traditional pasta instead of zoodles if you want a more filling dish.

Per serving (1 cup zucchini noodles and ½ chicken breast with sauce): Calories: 240; Total fat: 12g; Saturated fat: 2g; Carbohydrates: 16g; Sugar: 2g; Fiber: 2g; Protein: 16g

LEMON-THYME PORK TENDERLOIN

Serves 4 to 5 • **Prep time:** 5 MINUTES, PLUS 1 HOUR
TO MARINATE • **Cook time:** 45 MINUTES

GDM-Friendly | Lactation Support | Postpartum Recovery

This pork tenderloin is the ultimate "set it and forget it" meal. With little preparation, you can have a nourishing and protein-packed dish.

1 pound pork
  tenderloin, trimmed

Juice of 1 lemon

2 tablespoons extra-
  virgin olive oil

1 tablespoon minced
  garlic

1 teaspoon salt

⅛ teaspoon freshly
  ground black pepper

1 tablespoon fresh
  thyme leaves, or
  1 teaspoon dried
  thyme

1. Pierce the tenderloin with a fork and place it in a 9-by-12-inch baking dish.

2. In a medium bowl, whisk together the lemon juice, oil, garlic, salt, pepper, and thyme. Pour it over the tenderloin, then cover and refrigerate for at least 1 hour.

3. Preheat the oven to 375°F.

4. Remove the marinated tenderloin from the baking dish. Discard the marinade and place the tenderloin back in the dish.

5. Roast for 35 minutes, or until the internal temperature of the pork reads 145°F.

MAKE IT EASIER: The tenderloin can be marinated for up to 24 hours before cooking. Serve with a baked potato and a side salad for a balanced meal.

Per serving (3 ounces): Calories: 190; Total fat: 9g; Saturated fat: 2g; Carbohydrates: 1g; Sugar: <1g; Fiber: <1g; Protein: 24g

ROASTED CAULIFLOWER TACOS

Makes 8 tacos • Prep time: 15 MINUTES • Cook time: 20 MINUTES

Constipation Aid | Energy Booster | GDM-Friendly | Lactation Support

One-Pot | Postpartum Recovery

Cauliflower tacos are one of the best and most delicious ways to include this nutritional powerhouse in your diet. Cauliflower has key nutrients like vitamin C, choline, fiber, antioxidants—and the list goes on and on. Add this meatless taco to your rotation to keep your fiber intake up.

Cooking spray

1 head cauliflower, cut into florets

½ red onion, sliced

1 tablespoon low-sodium taco seasoning

2 tablespoons extra-virgin olive oil

5 ounces 2 percent plain Greek yogurt

½ tablespoon minced garlic

Juice of ½ lime

Pinch salt

8 (6-inch) corn or whole-grain tortillas

Sliced purple cabbage, for garnish (optional)

1. Preheat the oven to 425°F. Lightly coat the surface of a baking sheet with cooking spray.

2. In a medium bowl, combine the cauliflower and onion. Add the taco seasoning and oil and toss to coat.

3. Spread the seasoned cauliflower and onion in an even layer on the baking sheet and bake for 20 minutes.

4. Meanwhile, in a small bowl, combine the yogurt, garlic, lime, and salt.

5. Put the tortillas on a microwave-safe dish and cover them with a damp paper towel. Heat on high for 20 seconds, or until warm.

6. To serve, top each tortilla with the cauliflower filling, a dollop of Greek yogurt sauce, and purple cabbage slices (if using).

VARIATION TIP: If you are craving shrimp tacos, add cooked shrimp to increase healthy fats and protein. Use any leftover cauliflower filling as a side dish or as a topping for the Vegan Buddha Bowl (page 85).

Per serving (2 tacos): Calories: 242; Total fat: 9g; Saturated fat: 2g; Carbohydrates: 33g; Sugar: 6g; Fiber: 6g; Protein: 9g

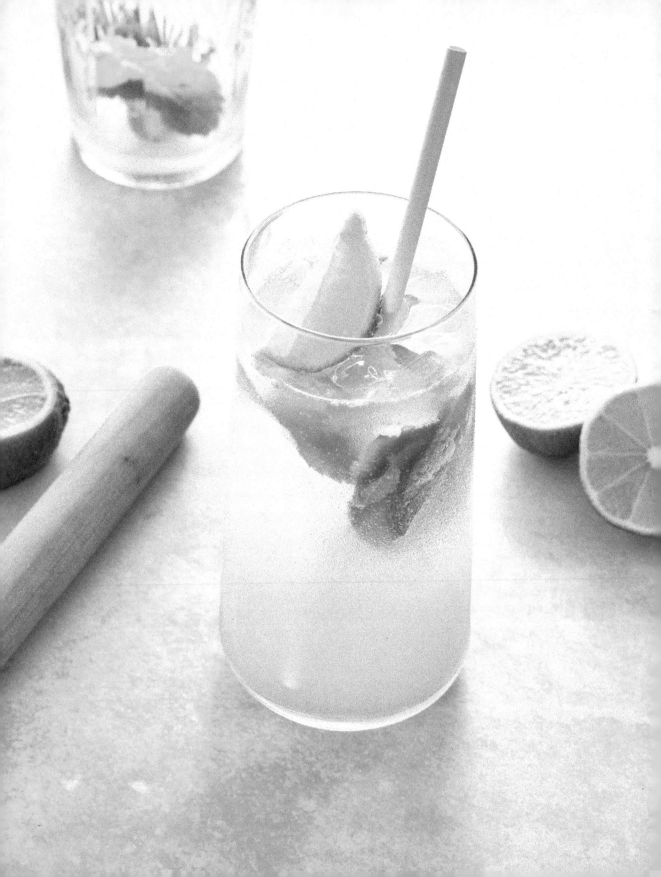

SEVEN

DESSERTS AND DRINKS

< COCONUT-MINT MOJITO
MOCKTAIL (PAGE 102)

GINGER LEMON SHOT

Makes 2 shots • Prep time: 10 MINUTES

Energy Booster | Nausea Relief | Quick

Ginger is the quintessential remedy for nausea. This shot packs the benefits of ginger in one quick shot, so you can get on with your day.

¼ cup ginger root, peeled and roughly chopped

⅓ cup freshly squeezed lemon juice

¼ cup coconut water

Pinch cayenne pepper

1. In a blender, combine the ginger, lemon juice, coconut water, and cayenne pepper and blend until smooth.

2. Strain the liquid through a fine-mesh strainer.

3. Pour the strained liquid into shot glasses and drink immediately.

MAKE IT EASIER: If drinking it doesn't work for you, try freezing the mixture in an ice-pop mold for a cool snack.

Per serving (¼ cup): Calories: 30; Total fat: <1g; Saturated fat: 0g; Carbohydrates: 7g; Sugar: 3g; Fiber: <1g; Protein: <1g

FIZZY CITRUS COOLER

This mocktail is packed with a variety of citrus juices, so it's full of important nutrients like vitamin C, folate, thiamin, and antioxidants. Enjoy this drink on a warm summer day poolside for a hydrating and satisfying sip.

1 teaspoon agave nectar

1 cup 100 percent pure orange juice

½ cup freshly squeezed lime juice

½ cup freshly squeezed lemon juice

1 (1-liter) bottle club soda

1 cup ice, plus more for serving

Orange, lime, and lemon slices, for garnish

1. In a tall pitcher or punch bowl, combine the agave nectar and orange, lime, and lemon juices. Stir in the club soda. Add the ice and stir until cold.

2. To serve, pour the cooler over ice, filling each glass. Include citrus slices as a garnish.

SUBSTITUTION TIP: For a lighter drink, add more club soda. Make ahead by prepping and storing the cooler mix, then add the ice and club soda just before serving.

Per serving (¾ cup): Calories: 24; Total fat: <1g; Saturated fat: 0g; Carbohydrates: 6g; Sugar: 4g; Fiber: <1g; Protein: <1g

COCONUT-MINT MOJITO MOCKTAIL

Serves 1 • **Prep time:** 5 MINUTES

Lactation Support | Postpartum Recovery | Quick

Who says you can't enjoy a fun and refreshing cocktail while you're pregnant? This mocktail is inspired by the classic mojito with a fun coconut twist. Bonus? This drink is super hydrating!

12 mint leaves, divided

1 tablespoon freshly squeezed lime juice

1 teaspoon pure maple syrup

½ cup coconut water

1 tablespoon unsweetened coconut milk

1 cup ice, divided

¼ cup lime seltzer

1. In a shaker, muddle 8 mint leaves with the lime juice.

2. Add the maple syrup, coconut water, coconut milk, and ½ cup of ice. Shake vigorously.

3. Put 4 mint leaves at the bottom of a highball glass and fill with the remaining ½ cup of ice. Strain the mixture from the shaker into the glass. Slowly pour the seltzer on top of the drink and serve.

Per serving (1 cup): Calories: 46; Total fat: <1g; Saturated fat: <1g; Carbohydrates: 11g; Sugar: 8g; Fiber: <1g; Protein: <1g

COCONUT HOT CHOCOLATE

Serves 4 • **Prep time:** 10 MINUTES • **Cook time:** 5 MINUTES

Energy Booster | Postpartum Recovery | Quick | Swelling Relief | Lactation Support

Some days call for a cozy cup of hot chocolate. But many of the commercial varieties are loaded with preservatives and, frankly, junk. This version is made with natural and vegan-friendly ingredients like unsweetened cocoa powder and coconut milk, which helps it check many important boxes in a healthy pregnancy diet.

2 (13.5-ounce) cans unsweetened coconut milk

½ cup semisweet chocolate chips

¼ cup unsweetened cocoa powder

¼ cup pure maple syrup

1 tablespoon vanilla extract

Pinch salt

Coconut whipped cream or vegan marshmallow, for garnish (optional)

1. In a large pot, combine the coconut milk, chocolate chips, cocoa powder, maple syrup, vanilla, and salt. Simmer over medium-low heat, stirring often, for about 5 minutes. Do not let it boil.

2. Serve in 4 mugs and top with whipped cream (if using).

SUBSTITUTION TIP: To add more protein, swap out the coconut milk for 2 percent dairy milk. For a minty cocoa, add a drop of mint extract to the mix and top with crushed candy cane. Just remember that the candy will add sugar to your beverage.

Per serving (1 cup): Calories: 494; Total fat: 40g; Saturated fat: 33g; Carbohydrates: 40g; Sugar: 32g; Fiber: 5g; Protein: 5g

CHEESECAKE-STUFFED STRAWBERRIES

Serves 3 to 5 • Prep time: 10 MINUTES

Energy Booster | GDM-Friendly | Lactation Support
Nausea Relief | Postpartum Recovery | Quick

Strawberries are one of the best sources of vitamin C, a nutrient that helps support the immune system and skin integrity. If you are craving cheesecake, these snacks will give you the satisfaction of that delicacy with more pregnancy-friendly nutrients.

1 (8-ounce) package cream cheese, softened

1 teaspoon stevia granules

¼ teaspoon vanilla extract

1 pound large strawberries

¼ cup graham cracker crumbs

2 tablespoons ground flaxseed

1. In a mixing bowl, beat the cream cheese, stevia, and vanilla until creamy.

2. Transfer the cream cheese mixture to a plastic storage bag. Snip off the corner of the bag and fill the strawberries with the cheesecake mixture.

3. In a small bowl, combine graham cracker crumbs and flaxseed, then sprinkle it on top of the filled strawberries.

SUBSTITUTION TIP: This recipe calls for stevia, which some people don't like or are allergic to. Simply use any sweetener you like if you can't use stevia.

MAKE IT EASIER: Store the filled strawberries covered in the refrigerator for up to 1 day.

Per serving (4 stuffed strawberries): Calories: 371; Total fat: 29g; Saturated fat: 16g; Carbohydrates: 23g; Sugar: 12g; Fiber: 5g; Protein: 8g

BLACK BEAN BROWNIES

Makes 10 brownies • Prep time: 5 MINUTES • Cook time: 20 MINUTES

Constipation Relief | Energy Booster | GDM-Friendly | Postpartum Recovery

When the sweet tooth strikes, these brownies will hit the spot! The fiber and protein in black beans will help you feel full longer than traditional brownies. And you won't even be able to taste the difference.

Cooking spray

1 (15-ounce) can black beans, rinsed and drained

2 tablespoons unsweet-ened cocoa powder

½ cup quick oats

Pinch salt

⅓ cup pure maple syrup

¼ cup coconut oil

1 teaspoon vanilla extract

½ teaspoon baking powder

1. Preheat the oven to 350°F. Lightly coat the interior of an 8-inch square baking dish with cooking spray.

2. In a food processor, combine the black beans, cocoa powder, oats, salt, maple syrup, coconut oil, vanilla, and baking powder and process until smooth. Pour the batter into the prepared baking dish.

3. Bake for 17 minutes, or until cooked through. Let cool before eating.

VARIATION TIP: For extra indulgence, stir in choco-late chips or peanut butter chips.

Per serving (1 brownie): Calories: 137; Total fat: 6g; Saturated fat: 5g; Carbohydrates: 18g; Sugar: 7g; Fiber: 4g; Protein: 3g

CHOCOLATE CRANBERRY BARK

Makes 25 to 32 pieces • Prep time: 5 MINUTES, PLUS
1 HOUR TO SET **• Cook time:** 2 MINUTES

Energy Booster | Freezer-Friendly | Nausea Relief

Chocolate cravings and pregnancy can go hand in hand. So why not make some homemade chocolate bark that also has nutritious ingredients? Dark chocolate contains magnesium that may help combat leg cramps, and the cranberries provide antioxidants.

2 cups dark chocolate chips

1 teaspoon coconut oil

¼ cup crushed walnuts

¼ cup dried cranberries

1 teaspoon chia seeds

1. Line a baking sheet with parchment paper.

2. In a medium microwave-safe bowl, melt the dark chocolate chips for 2 minutes, stirring every 20 seconds.

3. Once the chocolate has melted, stir in the coconut oil.

4. Pour the melted chocolate and coconut oil mixture onto the parchment-lined baking sheet and spread in a very thin layer.

5. Evenly sprinkle the walnuts, cranberries, and chia seeds on top of the chocolate and refrigerate for about 1 hour or until set.

6. Once the bark has set, break it into pieces.

SUBSTITUTION TIP: Have fun with the toppings that you use for this recipe. Coconut flakes, dried blueberries, and even sea salt are all great options.

MAKE IT EASIER: Make this ahead of time to have on hand whenever a craving hits. It can be stored in an airtight container in the refrigerator for up to 5 days or in the freezer for up to 6 months.

Per serving (1 piece): Calories: 100; Total fat: 7g; Saturated fat: 4g; Carbohydrates: 8g; Sugar: 5g; Fiber: 2g; Protein: 1g

BAKED APPLES

Serves 4 • Prep time: 5 MINUTES • Cook time: 1 HOUR

Constipation Aid | Energy Booster | GDM-Friendly | Lactation Support
Nausea Relief | One-Pot | Postpartum Recovery | Swelling Relief

If you're a fan of apple pie, then this dish is for you. Keeping the skin on the apples gives this dish a fiber boost, and using apple juice as a sweetener means less added sugar in the recipe. This dish can be served warm or cold.

4 Honeycrisp apples, cored and thinly sliced

1 tablespoon freshly squeezed lemon juice

1½ teaspoons coconut oil

¼ cup organic cane sugar

1½ teaspoons pumpkin pie spice

1 tablespoon raisins

3 tablespoons apple juice

Pinch salt

1. Preheat the oven to 350°F.

2. In a 9-by-13-inch baking dish, combine the apples, lemon juice, coconut oil, sugar, pumpkin pie spice, raisins, apple juice, and salt. Toss to combine and cover with foil.

3. Bake for 50 minutes, uncover, and bake for another 10 minutes.

SUBSTITUTION TIP: For a tart version of this dish, use Granny Smith apples instead of Honeycrisp. If desired, serve with a small scoop of vanilla ice cream.

Per serving (1 baked apple): Calories: 191; Total fat: 2g; Saturated fat: 2g; Carbohydrates: 47g; Sugar: 38g; Fiber: 6g; Protein: 1g

COFFEE-FREE HAZELNUT FRAPPÉ

Serves 4 • Prep time: 5 MINUTES

Constipation Aid | Energy Booster | Lactation Support

Postpartum Recovery | Quick

If you have given up caffeine during pregnancy, you may be missing your frozen cup of joe. This caffeine-free drink is not only safe for pregnancy, but also it contains ingredients like fiber, potassium, and iron—which you won't typically find at your corner coffee shop.

3 cups 2 percent milk

½ cup hazelnuts

8 pitted Medjool dates

¼ cup cacao powder

1 teaspoon vanilla extract

4 cups ice

Pinch salt

In a blender, combine the milk, hazelnuts, dates, cacao powder, vanilla, ice, and salt and blend until smooth.

SUBSTITUTION TIP: For a dairy-free version, swap in a nondairy milk of your choice. For more of a smoothie-style drink, add a frozen banana into the mix. Freeze leftovers in an ice-pop mold for an icy treat the next day.

Per serving (about 1 cup): Calories: 364; Total fat: 15g; Saturated fat: 4g; Carbohydrates: 52g; Sugar: 42g; Fiber: 7g; Protein: 11g

OATMEAL COOKIES

Makes 18 cookies • Prep time: 15 MINUTES • Cook time: 10 MINUTES

Constipation Aid | Energy Booster | Freezer-Friendly

Lactation Support | Postpartum Recovery

When your inner cookie monster comes for a visit, try these cookies for a satisfying and nutritious treat. Bananas add natural sweetness without the extra sugar, and they give this snack a boost of potassium. Unlike traditional oatmeal cookies, these contain plant-based protein from the peanut butter to help keep you feeling satisfied.

1 cup mashed ripe bananas (about 3 small bananas)

½ cup unsalted natural creamy peanut butter

2 cups old-fashioned rolled oats

½ cup dark chocolate chips

¼ cup raisins

1. Preheat the oven to 350°F. Line 2 baking sheets with parchment paper.

2. In a large bowl, combine the bananas, peanut butter, oats, chocolate chips, and raisins. Stir until well combined.

3. Using a 1½-tablespoon scoop, form the cookie dough into balls, placing each onto a baking sheet about 2 inches apart.

4. Bake the cookies for 10 minutes, or until set.

5. Let the cookies cool completely before removing them from the baking sheets.

6. Store in an airtight container at room temperature for up to 5 days or in the freezer for up to 2 months.

MAKE IT EASIER: Unlike traditional cookies, these won't spread when they bake. If you want a flatter cookie, form them into the desired shape with your fingers before baking.

Per serving (2 cookies): Calories: 247; Total fat: 13g; Saturated fat: 4g; Carbohydrates: 29g; Sugar: 10g; Fiber: 4g; Protein: 7g

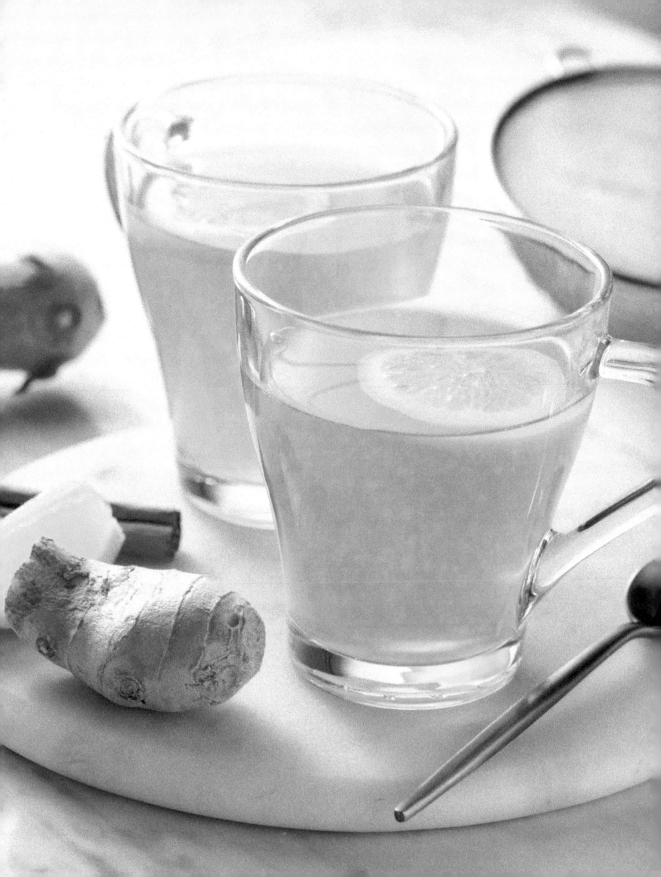

EIGHT

STAPLES AND EXTRAS

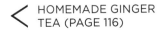

HOMEMADE GINGER
TEA (PAGE 116)

BONE BROTH

Makes 2 quarts • Prep time: 5 MINUTES • Cook time: 8 HOURS
GDM-Friendly | Freezer-Friendly | Nausea Relief | Postpartum Recovery

Bone broth is one of the greatest things to have on hand for soup bases or a sippable snack. Loaded with amino acids that help support your baby's growing and developing organs (as well as your stretching skin), this soup belongs in any pregnancy diet. Once your baby is born, the amino acids in this broth may help with postpartum healing.

3 pounds chicken or beef bones

2 tablespoons extra-virgin olive oil

1 cup white wine vinegar

12 cups water

2 bay leaves

3 carrots, peeled and halved

1 tablespoon freshly ground black pepper

Salt

1. Preheat the oven to 400°F. Line a baking sheet with parchment paper.

2. Arrange the bones on the baking sheet and drizzle the oil over them.

3. Roast the bones for 30 minutes.

4. Transfer the bones to a heavy stockpot. Add the vinegar, water, bay leaves, carrots, and pepper. Season with salt, then bring to a boil over high heat.

5. Once the water is boiling, reduce the heat to low. Simmer uncovered for at least 8 hours. Skim off any foam that appears at the surface of the broth.

6. Strain the broth.

7. Store the broth in an airtight container in the refrigerator for up to 1 week or in the freezer for up to 6 months.

MAKE IT EASIER: When you roast a whole chicken or have bone-in chicken for dinner, save the bones and use them for this broth.

Per serving (1 cup): Calories: 86; Total fat: 6g; Saturated fat: 2g; Carbohydrates: 1g; Sugar: 1g; Fiber: <1g; Protein: 4g

SPAGHETTI SAUCE

Makes 2 cups • Prep time: 5 MINUTES • Cook time: 45 MINUTES

GDM-Friendly | Freezer-Friendly | Nausea Relief | Postpartum Recovery

Spaghetti sauce deserves to be within reach in everyone's home because it is so great for jazzing up pasta, chicken, and many other dishes. Unfortunately, many premade sauces are loaded with sodium, added sugars, and even high-fructose corn syrup. This sauce contains pregnancy-friendly ingredients and is super simple to make. Enjoy it on your next spaghetti night!

1 (28-ounce) can whole peeled tomatoes

1 medium yellow onion, peeled and halved

2 tablespoons minced garlic

2 tablespoons extra-virgin olive oil

1 teaspoon dried oregano

1 teaspoon dried basil

1 bay leaf

Pinch red pepper flakes

1. In a medium, heavy-bottomed saucepan, combine the tomatoes with their juices, onion, garlic, oil, oregano, basil, bay leaf, and red pepper flakes (if using).

2. Bring the sauce to a simmer over medium-high heat, then reduce the heat to medium-low. Keep the sauce at a slow, steady simmer for about 45 minutes, stirring occasionally. Using a wooden spoon, crush the tomatoes against the side of the pot until your desired consistency is achieved.

3. Remove the pot from the heat and discard the onion and bay leaf.

MAKE IT EASIER: Make this sauce in double or triple batches, so you always have some on hand. It will keep in the refrigerator for up to 4 days, or in the freezer for up to 6 months.

Per serving (½ cup): Calories: 123; Total fat: 7g; Saturated fat: 1g; Carbohydrates: 12g; Sugar: 6g; Fiber: 2g; Protein: 2g

HOMEMADE RANCH DRESSING

Makes about ½ cup • Prep time: 5 MINUTES

GDM-Friendly | Quick

Ranch dressing goes with—well, just about everything! Instead of relying on the high-fat store-bought versions full of empty calories, whip up your own in a jiffy.

½ cup 2 percent plain Greek yogurt

1 teaspoon garlic powder

1½ teaspoons apple cider vinegar

½ teaspoon chopped fresh chives

Pinch salt

2 tablespoons water

In a medium bowl, combine the yogurt, garlic powder, vinegar, chives, salt, and water. Mix well.

SUBSTITUTION TIP: If you don't have fresh chives on hand, dried chives or dill both work well.

Per serving (1 tablespoon): Calories: 13; Total fat: <1g; Saturated fat: <1g; Carbohydrates: 1g; Sugar: 1g; Fiber: 0g; Protein: 2g

CHICKEN BROTH

Makes 6 quarts • Prep time: 15 MINUTES • Cook time: 1 HOUR

Freezer-Friendly | GDM-Friendly | Nausea Relief | One-Pot | Postpartum Recovery

Making your own chicken broth is surprisingly easy and ensures that you aren't eating anything you don't want while on your pregnancy diet. If you are feeling nauseated, homemade chicken broth hits the spot and can help balance electrolytes in a natural way.

2 tablespoons extra-virgin olive oil

2 medium onions, diced

2 carrots, peeled and cut crosswise into ¼-inch coins

6 pounds chicken legs and thighs, trimmed, cut into 2-inch pieces

6 quarts water

1 tablespoon salt

4 bay leaves

1. In a large heavy-bottomed pot, heat the oil over medium-high heat for 2 minutes, or until sizzling. Add the onion, carrots, and chicken and sauté for 7 minutes, or until the chicken is no longer pink.

2. Reduce the heat to low, cover, and cook for about 20 minutes.

3. Increase the heat to high and add the water, salt, and bay leaves.

4. Once the water starts boiling, immediately reduce the heat to low again, cover, and simmer for 30 minutes.

5. Strain and discard the solids and skim the fat before enjoying.

VARIATION TIP: If you are craving chicken and rice soup, add plain cooked rice after you strain the broth, then simmer for 10 minutes.

MAKE IT EASIER: You can leave the chicken, carrots, and onion in the soup if you want a hearty soup rather than a broth.

Per serving (1 cup): Calories: 45; Total fat: 2g; Saturated fat: 1g; Carbohydrates: 1g; Sugar: <1g; Fiber: <1g; Protein: 5g

HOMEMADE GINGER TEA

Makes 2 cups • Prep time: 5 MINUTES • Cook time: 10 MINUTES

GDM-Friendly | Lactation Support | Nausea Relief | One-Pot | Quick | Swelling Relief

Ginger tea is the ultimate go-to for nausea relief. Since some tea bags may contain unsavory additions (like microplastics), making your own is one way to ensure that what you are putting in your body is the healthiest option for both you and your baby.

2-inch chunk fresh ginger, cut into pieces

2 cups water

1 cinnamon stick

Lemon wedge, for serving

1. In a small saucepan, combine the ginger, water, and cinnamon stick and bring to a boil over high heat.

2. Once boiling, reduce the heat to low and simmer for 5 minutes.

3. Remove the pot from the heat. Strain the mixture through a fine-mesh sieve into a mug.

4. Squeeze the juice from one lemon wedge into the tea before serving.

SUBSTITUTION TIP: This tea can be enjoyed iced as well. Simply pour the tea over a cup of ice (in a heat-resistant cup!) and sip away.

Per serving (1 cup): Calories: 2; Total fat: 0g; Saturated fat: 0g; Carbohydrates: <1g; Sugar: 0g; Fiber: 0g; Protein: 0g

HONEY MUSTARD SAUCE

Makes about 1 cup • **Prep time:** 4 MINUTES

One-Pot | Quick

Honey mustard can be loaded with added sugar, high-fat ingredients, and artificial colors. This pregnancy-friendly version offers up protein, calcium, and live probiotics, thanks to the Greek yogurt. This condiment goes well with many dishes as a dip, side, or spread.

½ cup 2 percent plain Greek yogurt

¼ cup extra-virgin olive oil

¼ cup Dijon mustard

3 tablespoons honey

2 tablespoons freshly squeezed lemon juice

1 teaspoon garlic powder

Salt

Freshly ground black pepper

In a small dish, combine the yogurt, oil, mustard, honey, lemon juice, garlic powder, salt, and pepper. Whisk until smooth.

MAKE IT EASIER: Cover any leftovers and store in the refrigerator for up to 4 days.

Per serving (1 tablespoon): Calories: 52; Total fat: 4g; Saturated fat: 1g; Carbohydrates: 4g; Sugar: 4g; Fiber: <1g; Protein: 1g

CHIA ZINGER

If constipation has graced you with its presence, downing one of these drinks may help get things moving in the right direction. Try this refreshing, fiber-packed zinger and hopefully you will be feeling a bit better in no time.

1 cup cold water

½ tablespoon chia seeds

Juice of ½ lime

¼ teaspoon pure maple syrup

Pinch salt

1. In a glass, combine the water, chia seeds, lime juice, maple syrup, and salt. Stir well.

2. Let the mixture sit for 15 minutes at room temperature to allow time for the seeds to hydrate and begin to gel.

3. Stir again to prevent the chia seeds from settling to the bottom of the glass, and drink immediately.

VARIATION TIP: Add orange juice, grapefruit juice, or lemon juice for different flavors and more nutritional value.

Per serving (1 cup): Calories: 40; Total fat: 2g; Saturated fat: 0g; Carbohydrates: 6g; Sugar: 1g; Fiber: 2g; Protein: 1g

BELLY BUTTER

Rubbing your growing belly with belly butter can be a decadent and soothing experience, especially once your skin starts stretching. And while using belly butter every day won't guarantee that you won't get stretch marks, it certainly won't hurt.

½ cup cocoa butter

1 tablespoon coconut oil

½ teaspoon extra-virgin olive oil

1. In a double boiler, heat the cocoa butter, coconut oil, and olive oil over medium heat for 5 minutes, stirring occasionally with a wooden spoon, until both the cocoa butter and coconut oil have melted.

2. Remove from the heat and transfer to a jar.

3. Allow to cool completely (at least 25 minutes) before using.

SUBSTITUTION TIP: Add 5 drops of lavender or a citrus essential oil in step 2 and stir well before transferring to the jar. If you are sensitive to essential oils, do not include them. Note that certain essential oils should be avoided during pregnancy, so always check with your health-care provider before you make any additions.

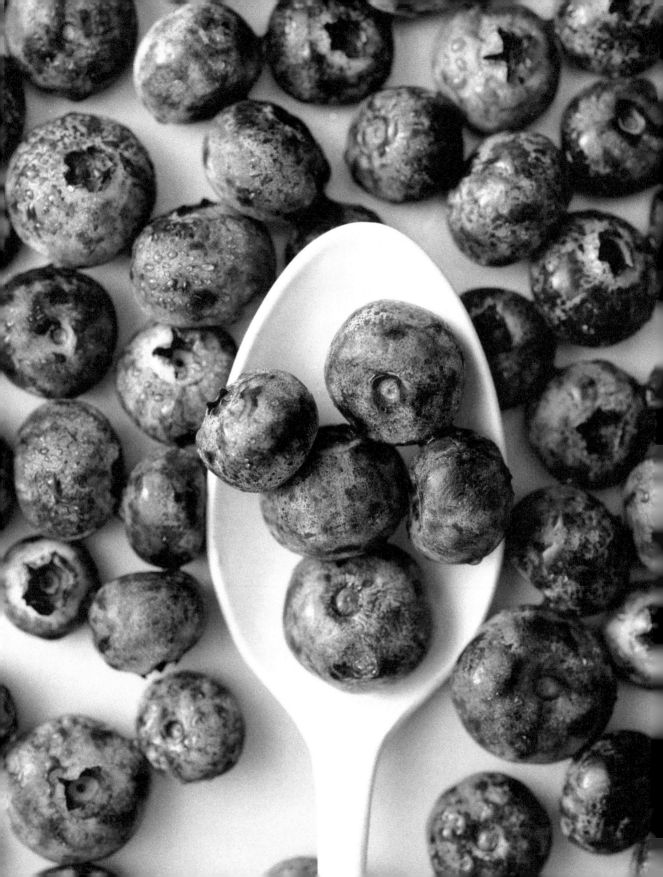

MEASUREMENT CONVERSIONS

VOLUME EQUIV.	US STANDARD	US STANDARD (OUNCES)	METRIC (APPROX.)
LIQUID	2 tablespoons	1 fl. oz.	30 mL
	¼ cup	2 fl. oz.	60 mL
	½ cup	4 fl. oz.	120 mL
	1 cup	8 fl. oz.	240 mL
	1½ cups	12 fl. oz.	355 mL
	2 cups or 1 pint	16 fl. oz.	475 mL
	4 cups or 1 quart	32 fl. oz.	1 L
	1 gallon	128 fl. oz.	4 L
DRY	⅛ teaspoon	—	0.5 mL
	¼ teaspoon	—	1 mL
	½ teaspoon	—	2 mL
	¾ teaspoon	—	4 mL
	1 teaspoon	—	5 mL
	1 tablespoon	—	15 mL
	¼ cup	—	59 mL
	⅓ cup	—	79 mL
	½ cup	—	118 mL
	⅔ cup	—	156 mL
	¾ cup	—	177 mL
	1 cup	—	235 mL
	2 cups or 1 pint	—	475 mL
	3 cups	—	700 mL
	4 cups or 1 quart	—	1 L
	½ gallon	—	2 L
	1 gallon	—	4 L

WEIGHT EQUIVALENTS

US STANDARD	METRIC (APPROX.)
½ ounce	15 g
1 ounce	30 g
2 ounces	60 g
4 ounces	115 g
8 ounces	225 g
12 ounces	340 g
16 ounces or 1 pound	455 g

OVEN TEMPERATURES

FAHRENHEIT	CELSIUS (APPROX.)
250°F	120°C
300°F	150°C
325°F	165°C
350°F	180°C
375°F	190°C
400°F	200°C
425°F	220°C
450°F	230°C

RESOURCES

Academy of Nutrition and Dietetics
EatRight.org/health/pregnancy/what-to-eat-when-expecting
/eating-right-during-pregnancy

The American College of Obstetrics and Gynecologists
ACOG.org/womens-health/resources-for-you?utm_source=redirect&utm
_medium=web&utm_campaign=otn#f:@patientportalcontenttype=[faqs]

March of Dimes
MarchOfDimes.org/index.aspx

United States Department of Agriculture, MyPlate
MyPlate.gov/life-stages/pregnancy-and-breastfeeding

**US Department of Health and Human Services,
Office on Women's Health**
WomensHealth.gov/pregnancy

REFERENCES

Jouanne, Marie, Sarah Oddoux, Antoine Noël, and Anne Sophie Voisin-Chiret. "Nutrient Requirements during Pregnancy and Lactation." *Nutrients* 13, no. 2 (February 21, 2021): 692. doi.org/10.3390/nu13020692.

Korsmo, Hunter W., Xinyin Jiang, and Marie A. Caudill. "Choline: Exploring the Growing Science on Its Benefits for Moms and Babies." *Nutrients* 11, no. 8: 1823 (August 7, 2019): 1823. doi.org/10.3390/nu11081823.

Lian, Rui-Han, Ping-An Qi, Tao Yuan, Pei-Jiing Yan, Wen-Wen Qiu, Ying Wei, Ya-Guang Hu, Ke-Hu Yang, and Bin Yi. "Systematic Review and Meta-Analysis of Vitamin D Deficiency in Different Pregnancy on Preterm Birth: Deficiency in Middle Pregnancy Might Be at Risk." *Medicine* 100, no. 24 (June 18, 2021): e26303. doi.org/10.1097/MD.0000000000026303.

Martinat, Maud, Moïra Rossitto, Mathieu Di Miceli, and Sophie Layé. "Perinatal Dietary Polyunsaturated Fatty Acids in Brain Development, Role in Neurodevelopmental Disorders." *Nutrients* 13, no 4 (April 2, 2021): 1185. doi.org/10.3390/nu13041185.

Patti, Marisa A., Nan Li, Melissa Eliot, Craig Newschaffer, Kimberly Yolton, Jane Khoury, Aimin Chen, et al. "Association between Self-Reported Caffeine Intake During Pregnancy and Social Responsiveness Scores in Childhood: The EARLI and HOME Studies." *PLoS One* 16, no. 1 (January 15, 2021): e0245079. doi.org/10.1371/journal.pone.0245079.

Prasad, Priya, Mari Mori, Helga V. Toriello, and ACMG Professional Practice and Guidelines Committee. "Focused Revision: Policy Statement on Folic Acid and Neural Tube Defects." *Genetics in Medicine* (July 6, 2021). doi.org/10.1038/s41436-021-01226-6.

Van Dael, Peter. "Role of N-3 Long-Chain Polyunsaturated Fatty Acids in Human Nutrition and Health: Review of Recent Studies and Recommendations." *Nutrition Research and Practice* 15, no. 2 (April 2021): 137–159. doi.org/10.4162/nrp.2021.15.2.137.

SYMPTOM INDEX

SWELLING RELIEF

INDEX

Acknowledgments

A hearty thank-you is due to so many people who helped me throughout this cookbook journey.

A special acknowledgment has to go to Erin Davis, who held my hand throughout the entire process. Your words of encouragement and advice helped shape this cookbook in an amazing way.

I would like to thank Mary Grace Gilkey for being such a help during the recipe development phase. I enjoyed being your preceptor during your time at the Medical University of South Carolina, and I appreciate all of your creativity and hard work.

And to my family and colleagues who were my ever-present cheerleaders—your support means the world to me.

And finally, to all of the pregnant people out there who are looking for some reliable nutrition information, you were my inspiration, and I hope this book helps make your journey a bit less stressful and a tad more delicious.

About the Author

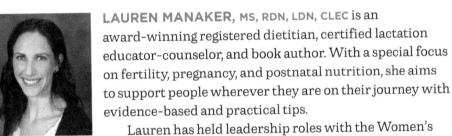

LAUREN MANAKER, MS, RDN, LDN, CLEC is an award-winning registered dietitian, certified lactation educator-counselor, and book author. With a special focus on fertility, pregnancy, and postnatal nutrition, she aims to support people wherever they are on their journey with evidence-based and practical tips.

Lauren has held leadership roles with the Women's Health Dietetic Practice Group of the Academy of Nutrition and Dietetics and has been featured in many media outlets, including *U.S. News and World Report*, *Scary Mommy*, *Women's Health*, CNN, and more. As a consultant for healthy food and supplement brands, she has helped create prenatal supplements and many other products that support the lactation journey. This is her second pregnancy-focused cookbook.

When she is not working, Lauren is likely on the water enjoying all that her home state of South Carolina has to offer with her young daughter, husband, and rescue pup. Find her on Instagram at @LaurenLovesNutrition.

CPSIA information can be obtained
at www.ICGtesting.com
Printed in the USA
JSHW030854250122
22214JS00002B/2